Opening Up

A GUIDE TO CREATING AND SUSTAINING
OPEN RELATIONSHIPS

Opening Up

A GUIDE TO CREATING AND SUSTAINING
OPEN RELATIONSHIPS

Tristan Taormino

CLEIS
PRESS

Published in the United States by Cleis Press Inc.,
P.O. Box 14697, San Francisco, California 94114.
Printed in the United States.
Cover design: Scott Idleman
Cover photograph: Glowimages/Getty Images
Book design: Karen Quigg
Cleis Press logo art: Juana Alicia
First Edition.
10 9

The case histories, quotes, and anecdotes in this book are true. They are all based on actual, voluntary interviews given for the purposes of this publication. However, names, locations, and other identifying material may have been changed to protect the identity of the subjects. Similarities in names or other physically descriptive characteristics between any of the subjects of this book and any other person is purely coincidental.

Some parts of Chapter 18 first appeared in *The Ultimate Guide to Anal Sex for Women*, by Tristan Taormino (San Francisco: Cleis Press, 2006).

Library of Congress Cataloging-in-Publication Data

Taormino, Tristan, 1971-
    Opening up : a guide to creating and sustaining open relationships / Tristan Taormino. — 1st ed.
        p. cm.
Includes bibliographical references.
ISBN 978-1-57344-295-4 (pbk. : alk. paper)
    1. Non-monogamous relationships. I. Title.

HQ980.T36 2008
306.84'23—dc22

                                        2008008653

I dedicate this book to
every person who has the courage
to live and love outside the box

Acknowledgments

I MUST ACKNOWLEDGE some of the pioneers in this field whose work has made it possible for mine to exist: Deborah Anapol, Joan and Larry Constantine, Dossie Easton and Janet Hardy, Raven Kaldera, Ronald Mazur, and Ryam Nearing. I had my first light-bulb moment about this topic at dinner with two friends after a panel discussion by Jill Carter, Queen Cougar, and Vi Johnson—they all unknowingly played a part in the early germination of the idea. Throughout the years, I have learned a great deal from classes about polyamory taught by Jon and Carin, Dossie Easton, Sarah Sloane, Anita Wagner, and Lolita Wolf. Several years ago, I worked jointly on a book proposal on this topic with Dr. Winston Wilde, and although we ended up not collaborating on the project, I am forever grateful to him for his knowledge, experience, mentoring, and love.

I would like to thank Jennifer Ferris of Kelsey Transcripts, Helen Boyd, and Emily Salzfass for their transcription work. Helen Boyd also provided invaluable research assistance. Tey Meadows assisted me in finding transcription help, located important legal articles, and sparked inspiration in me when it was greatly needed. Valerie White of the Sexual Freedom Legal Defense and Education Fund was generous with her time and wisdom. Mark Michaels and Patricia Johnson had a huge influence on this work; they shared rare books from their collection, discussed their experiences as Tantra and relationship coaches, and had innumerable conversations that helped me conceptualize key sections. Anita Wagner was an integral part of this book: she spread the word far and wide, distributed interviews, shared her insight, and on top of all that, single-handedly compiled the majority of the Resource Guide. Members of several LiveJournal communities helped get the word out as I searched for interviewees. The incredible people who make up the Dark Odyssey community inspire and teach me year after year.

My agent, Andrew Blauner, helped kick-start this project after it had been shelved and gathering dust. He is my cheerleader, my gentle reminder, my advocate, and my friend. Thanks to everyone at Cleis Press for their support. My publishers, Felice Newman and Frédérique Delacoste, accepted delays with grace and continue to be a joy to work with; Felice edited the manuscript herself and, as always, provided thoughtful, invaluable editorial advice.

My friends mean so much to me and have cheered me on in this project. Thanks to Arielle, Barb O'Neill and Dylan Bosseau, Clyde, Helen Boyd and Betty Crow, David Aguilar, Ira Levine and Nina Hartley, Kate Larkin and Johann vanOverbeek, Mark Michaels and Patricia Johnston, Mary DiStefano and Dana Wegener, Tey Meadows, Toni Amato and Opn. Thanks to my mother, who continues to support me unconditionally.

Many writers' partners feel "widowed" when the writer starts a new book. My partner, Colten Tognazzini, is no different and yet he was an unbelievable support to me. I literally could not have researched and written this book without him. He organized responses from my LiveJournal posting for interviewees; he rewired the phone line, set up the microphone, and figured out the software so I could record all my interviews on my laptop; he fed me so I could keep writing; he edited the bibliography; he allowed me the time and space to dive headfirst into the project and let it consume me; he listened while I bounced around ideas; he picked up the slack and ran our businesses so I could concentrate on the book; he made me take short breaks so I wouldn't go insane; he let me work until my brain was fried and my eyesight blurry, then he gently told me to put the computer down.

And finally, my undying gratitude goes to all the people I interviewed. They took time out of their busy lives to answer my written interview questions, and some took even more time to talk to me on the phone or in person. They were truly excited about the book and willing to talk about nearly anything and everything. Their candor and courage is amazing; what they said and how they said it was invaluable. I learned so much from every single one of them. Their words, their voices, their struggles, their opinions, their successes, and their challenges make this book what it is.

Contents

Opening Up to the Possibilities: Challenging Monogamy and Revolutionizing Relationships

MY LIFE'S WORK for more than a decade has been dedicated to educating and empowering people around their sexuality. I write about sex, I teach workshops and lecture about sex, I answer people's questions about sex, I demonstrate techniques for sex, I make sex-positive movies, and I produce sex events. Because of my work and my never-ending interest in all things sexual, I have witnessed and indulged in a wide variety of sexual experiences and met people from all walks of life. I've met people who are straight, queer, bi, vanilla, kinky, and just plain horny. I've made friends with leatherfolk, swingers, gender-queers, sex workers, polyamorous people, Tantra practitioners, Pagans, and sex radicals.

The first time I saw someone have sex right in front of me, I was mesmerized, awestruck, turned on. It was really cool. The 400th time, it's still cool, but it's different. I found myself less interested in the surface of what I was seeing—how he licks her, the noises she makes when she fucks her, the way he looks when she plays with his ass, what he says when he talks dirty to him, and on and on. Instead, I was much more fascinated by who the people are. Are they a couple? How long have they been together? What made them decide to come to this sex event? What do they like about having public sex? Who is that other woman I often see making out with them both? Do they have sex with other people? I want to know what the context is for what I am watching. I want to know about the inner workings of their relationship.

And it was no wonder. As I got to know these people, I discovered that their relationships were a lot more intriguing, complex, and transgressive than their sex lives (and their sex lives were pretty amazing). In addition to sharp communication skills and a creative sense of identity, they all appeared to have one thing in common: they were all in nonmonogamous relationships. And they'd found a way to make those relationships work so well that they exuded an above-average level of sexual and emotional satisfaction—something that in my experience and observation seems to elude a lot of people. So, I wondered, just how do they do it?

The Decline of Marriage and Monogamy

> *Most of the world's peoples, throughout history and around the globe, have arranged things so that marriage and sexual exclusivity are not the same thing.* —The Myth of Monogamy[1]

It's no secret that traditional monogamous marriage in America is in serious trouble and has been for quite a while. The model of the stay-at-home wife and the husband as sole breadwinner began to change during the Industrial Revolution; it shifted significantly when women entered the workforce in record numbers during World War II. Once women began working outside the home, earning their own money (albeit less money for the same work), exploring education and career opportunities, gender roles shifted and marriage changed. In the 1950s there was a brief return to more traditional coupling: 96 percent of people of childbearing age were married, and they got married at a younger age.[2] This period in what I call "*Leave It to Beaver* Land" didn't last for very long. The 1960s brought the sexual revolution, part of a counterculture movement among young people that openly questioned prevailing norms about sex and gender. Through writing, activist groups, and public demonstrations, men and women critiqued the Vietnam War, capitalism, and the nuclear family. They promoted sexual liberation and "free love" over monogamy and marriage. Along with this change in cultural ideas and social norms came a decline in marriage rates, an increase in divorce rates, and a decrease in the number of children people had.[3]

The activism of the sixties gave birth to the women's movement, which mobilized women and men to challenge gender roles, stereotypes, and inequality. Access to birth control and legalized abortion meant women could take charge of their reproductive choices and have sex for pleasure, not just for procreation. Feminists critiqued and rejected marriage as a patriarchal institution. In 1970, the marriage rate briefly increased, but divorce rates showed a sizable increase, too: 14.9 per 1,000 married women age 15 and older, up from 9.2 in 1960. By 1975, the marriage rate began to decline again and divorce rates continued to rise.[4] The seventies also saw a burst of academic work on swingers and alternative relationships and the publication of over a dozen books on those subjects. The Stonewall Riots of 1969 jump-started the gay and lesbian civil rights movement, giving traditional marriage and nuclear families yet another detractor: queer people.

In the eighties, marriage rates continued to drop. Part of the decline was blamed on the rise of another form of coupling: unmarried heterosexual couples who lived together (and were given the decidedly unsexy moniker "cohabitators"). Although cohabitators weren't new, by the eighties there were enough of them that sociologists and the US Census Bureau began to take notice. Divorce rates kept rising in the eighties until 1995, when they began to decline slightly, although not as quickly as marriage rates did. By the nineties, more gay, lesbian, bisexual, and transgendered people were coming out of the closet than ever before. They were living together, having commitment ceremonies, and raising children; the greater visibility of this community continued to redefine ideas about relationships and family.

In 2004, the marriage rate was 39.9 per 1,000 unmarried women age 15 and older, which means that in less than 50 years, the rate had dropped nearly 50 percent.[5] In the same time period, rates for second, third, and fourth marriages increased, although those marriages don't necessarily fare any better: statistics show that the divorce rate for remarriages is even higher than for first marriages.[6] Clearly, the structure, expectations, and functionality of marriage are not as desirable or functional as they were 50 years ago.

There's another significant indicator that monogamous marriages and relationships aren't working: cheating is epidemic. The Kinsey Report was the first to offer statistics on the subject from a large study published in 1953; it reported that 26 percent of wives and 50 percent of husbands had at least one affair by the time they were 40 years old. Other studies followed, with similar findings. According to the *Janus Report* of 1993, more than one-third of men and more than one-quarter of women admit to having had at least one extramarital sexual experience. Forty percent of divorced women and 45 percent of divorced men reported having had more than one extramarital sexual relationship while they were still married.[7] In a 2007 poll conducted by MSNBC and iVillage, half of more than 70,000 respondents said they've been unfaithful at some point in their lives, and 22 percent have cheated on their current partner.[8]

While nearly anyone you ask will tell you cheating is wrong and immoral, research obviously reflects decidedly different behavior.

Having an affair has become like a shadow institution in this country: it's so ingrained in our culture that we take it for granted as inevitable. Cheating on one's partner is a pivotal plot point in countless television shows, movies, plays, operas, pop songs, and even commercials. It has become so widespread that it has spawned an entire industry of dating websites for cheaters to meet other cheaters, books and self-help programs, and private investigation services. Although publicly it's considered unacceptable, it has become an accepted part of life.

For those people who manage to avoid cheating (or being cheated on), there is still a general dissatisfaction with monogamous relationships. Complaints about being stuck in a rut abound. Everywhere you look, you are urged to "spice up" your sex life, reignite the romance, combat monotony, or bring back the spark in your relationship. The number of magazine articles, books, talk show episodes, workshops, retreats—not to mention people's individual counseling sessions—devoted to these topics is staggering.[9] Couples therapy is a booming business. Lots of people seem pretty unhappy.

Monogamy's Mythology

Those who talk most about the blessings of marriage and the constancy of its vows are the very people who declare that if the chain were broken and the prisoners left free to choose, the whole social fabric would fly asunder. You cannot have the argument both ways. If the prisoner is happy, why lock him in? If he is not, why pretend that he is? —George Bernard Shaw[10]

It's no wonder people are so dissatisfied: monogamy sets most people up to fail. The rules of traditional monogamy are clear: you've vowed to be emotionally and sexually exclusive with one person forever. But it's the unspoken rules that will trip you up. We've collectively been sold a fairy tale of finding that one person with whom you'll live happily ever after. The expectations are endless: your one-and-only is your soul mate, the person with whom you are 100 percent sexually and emotionally compatible, your "other half" with whom you share the same values about everything. He or she will fulfill all your needs—physical, emotional, psychological, affectionate, financial, romantic, sexual, and spiritual. If you are truly in love, you will never have any desire for anything from anyone else.

Some people see through this unspoken mythology, consciously reject the unreasonable expectations, decide to commit to one partner, and are satisfied. These folks *choose* monogamy and it works for them. But it is more common that people are monogamous not by choice, but by default; they believe monogamy is what everyone else is doing, what is expected, and how relationships are supposed to be. In addition, they have grown up with messages about the fairy tale, it has seeped into their consciousness, and they work hard to live up to all the hype. The problem is that those unspoken expectations of monogamy are unrealistic and unattainable.

When someone in a monogamous relationship is first confronted with a desire that contradicts the mythology, it causes a range of reactions. Perhaps you realize your partner isn't meeting all your needs. Or you find yourself attracted to someone else. At first you feel guilty because you're not supposed to have those feelings. They're supposed to be reserved for your one-and-only! If you were really in love… But you have them, and you have some options. You can recognize the feeling without shame or guilt and decide you're not going to act on it because you don't need to or want to. You will probably feel good about this decision—it is the decision made by people who've thought about monogamy and chosen it consciously. But the next three options are far more common: 1) Deny the desire: This is a coping mechanism that sends your feelings underground, where they fester, leading to resentment, anger, and disconnection from your partner. 2) Indulge the desire: Your only option here is to cheat, which leads to deception and betrayal. 3) Fulfill the desire:

You can only truly fulfill it if you end your current relationship and then start one with the new person. Serial monogamy, here we come!

In actuality, there is another option. There are several, in fact. But they all require that you give up monogamy. Cheaters do at least one honest thing: they acknowledge that one partner can't meet all their needs and that they want to have sex or a relationship with someone other than their current partner. Then they fuck everything up by lying. They act on their desire with dishonesty by sneaking around, keeping secrets, and shutting down communication with their partner.

Nonmonogamy as an Alternative Choice

If you love something, set it free. If it comes back to you, it's yours.
If it doesn't, it never was. —Anonymous

People who practice nonmonogamy begin from the same premise: one partner cannot meet all their needs and they may want to have sex or a relationship with someone other than their current partner. But instead of hiding it, they bring this fact out in the open. They don't stifle their behavior based on how they're supposed to act. They open the lines of communication. They talk honestly about what they want, face their fears and the fears of others, and figure out a way to pursue their desire without deception. They don't limit themselves to sharing affection, flirting, sex, connection, romance, and love with just one person. They believe strongly that you can have all these things with multiple people and do it in an ethical, responsible way.

There are no scripts or models for open relationships, so people in them must invent their partnerships by living them. When their relationships change, they are just as likely to renegotiate them to make them work as they are to end them. Because they have multiple experiences, people, and relationships in their life, they rarely get stuck in that rut that monogamous people complain about.

On the surface, it may seem that people in nonmonogamous relationships give up the comfort and security of monogamy. After all, on a regular basis they must confront one of our deepest fears—that a partner is going to leave. But they value their freedom and the freedom of their partners, and with that freedom comes, for some, a greater sense of security. It sounds like a contradiction, but one of the most profound things I have learned from people in nonmonogamous relationships is how confident and content they feel about the strength of their partnerships. One woman said she knows her partners are in a relationship because they want to be, not out of any obligation. Another told me that because her relationships aren't built on false ideas about exclusivity forever, she feels more cherished by her partners; she said, "There is an investment in what we have rather than what we should have." But all this freedom doesn't mean it's a free-for-all. Nonmonogamous folks are constantly engaged in their relationships: they negotiate and establish boundaries, respect them, test them, and, yes, even violate them. But the limits are not assumed or set by society; they are consciously chosen.

Who are these daring revolutionaries? When most people think of those with multiple partners, a few images come to mind. The cheating spouse and his mistress. Crazy swingers, wild orgies, and sex parties. Polygamous people of a foreign culture in a faraway land. But nonmonogamous people are not a strange or rare breed. They are everywhere, all around you. They belong to hip urban enclaves and they live on farms in rural America. They have high school diplomas and they have PhDs. They may have little in common in their everyday lives. What they share is the honesty and willingness to take a leap and create relationships that defy everything we've been taught.

My Research

In the past 10 years, I've studied a lot about polyamory and other forms of nonmonogamy. What always struck me, in reading books and attending workshops, was that how-to information is helpful, but it's just a framework. I can remember attending talks on the subject and walking away feeling that I didn't know any more than I did before. Polyamory was portrayed in an idealistic way where everyone was on the same page, having tons of sex and getting along great. It made me a little suspicious.

Several years ago, while out of town, I went to dinner with a friend and a woman I knew from the area. I knew both of them were polyamorous, and we struck up a conversation about it. My friend said, "My primary partner and I don't have a sexual relationship. We have sex with our other partners. But we are 100 percent committed to one another." I was surprised, because what she was saying contradicted all the models I knew. Our companion was a very high-profile leader in the BDSM community, and she'd been with her primary partner for a long time. "Della and I became poly after she cheated on me. I was sort of dragged into polyamory nonconsensually, in other words. When I found out she cheated, I was hurt and angry, but when I cooled down, I realized I did not want to end our relationship. So, we sat down and said, What can we do to make this work?"

What I realized that night, listening to their stories, was that I hadn't heard a lot of people talk about the specifics of their situations. When someone is willing to share the nitty-gritty details of their life, we can learn from their experiences. But people have to have the courage to tell the good, the bad, the ugly, the quirky, the embarrassing, so others know they are not alone.

That is why it was important to include as many different voices and versions of nonmonogamy as I could in this book. I have my own experiences with open relationships, both successful and unsuccessful. I've tried many different styles of nonmonogamy. I have been in my current open relationship for seven years. But I think it's useful to get as many different perspectives as possible about such a broad topic. So I turned to the people I knew who were coloring outside the lines of monogamy.

I created a written questionnaire and emailed it to personal contacts and leaders of local polyamory groups. In addition, I posted information about the questionnaire in online forums and encouraged people to forward and distribute the posting to others. It's a self-selecting group of people, or what researchers call a "snowball sample": I send the interview to people, they send it to partners and friends, and so on, like a chain letter. I'm not a sociologist—this is not a scientific study, and the participants are not a random sample—but the information is valuable nonetheless, especially since there is so little research about people in open relationships.

In total, I collected information from 126 respondents. I received written questionnaires from 121 of them. I did follow-up interviews with 80: 38 of them in person, 20 via email, and 22 by telephone. (Five of the 38 in-person interviewees did not complete the written questionnaire in advance; I collected their demographic information during the course of the interview.)

My study included 66 women, 50 men, and 10 people who identified as transgender or "other." Thirty-eight percent identified as bisexual, bi/queer, bi/straight, or bi/pansexual. Thirty-seven percent identified as straight or straight/bi; 19 percent as gay, lesbian, or queer; and 6 percent as pansexual or omnisexual. The youngest person was 21, the oldest was 72, and the average age was 37. The majority of respondents were white (about 80 percent). People came from 28 states and were pretty equally divided across the US: 30 percent from the South, 29 percent from the Northeast, 20 percent from the West, and 19 percent from the Midwest. Two participants were from Canada. The group included a food-service worker, a cosmetic sales representative, a Gaming Commission officer, a state tax auditor, a porn performer, an enlisted member of the Army, and a minister. The most common occupation was teaching, with six elementary, middle, and high school teachers and four professors. In some cases, I interviewed both partners of a couple or all members of a triad; in others, I obtained information from only one member, reflecting just that person's perspective of the relationship.

Reading *Opening Up*

This book is a window into the world of possibilities beyond monogamy. It's a study and a road map, a guidebook and a manifesto. Just by picking it up, you show some interest in the topic. Maybe you are curious about or considering an open relationship. Perhaps you have been polyamorous for most of your life and you're looking for advice about how to actively support your open relationship. You might be the loved one of a person in an open relationship who wants to better understand nonmonogamy, or a member of a helping profession (a doctor, therapist, or social worker) who needs to better understand it. I hope there is something useful here for all of you.

I had an important epiphany while putting this book together: there is no formula for an open relationship. Everyone does nonmonogamy differently. Each story and each relationship is unique. There are similarities and patterns, but no one does it exactly the same as anyone else. Consider the observations and advice in this book a guide for creating open relationships and making them work. Learn from the people I interviewed, who share their clarity and confusion, their heartbreak and joy, their struggles and success stories. Take it all in as you design your relationships, and remember: life is in the details.

The first section of the book is an introduction to open relationships. In Chapter 1, I cover a brief history of different forms of nonmonogamy since the 1950s and define important terms that are used throughout the book. Chapter 2 exposes and corrects myths about nonmonogamy. Why people choose open relationships is the subject of Chapter 3, and some of the principles that make them work are outlined in Chapter 4. The second section, Chapters 5 through 10, describes various styles of open relationships, including partnered nonmonogamy, swinging, polyamory, solo polyamory, polyfidelity, and mono/poly combinations. Beginning with Chapter 5 and continuing through Chapter 17, there is a more detailed look at one (or several) of the subjects I interviewed at the end of each chapter.

The third section of the book is your road map to creating and sustaining open relationships. Chapter 11 offers guidelines and exercises to help you design your ideal relationship. In Chapter 12, I dig into jealousy and its many companions, including envy, insecurity, possessiveness, and resentment. Chapter 13 delves into the concept of *compersion*, which has been called the opposite of jealousy. Some of the common challenges and conflicts people in open relationships must deal with—what happens when a partner gets into a new relationship, time management, miscommunication, and agreement violations—are explored in Chapter 14. Coping with change is the focus of Chapter 15. In Chapter 16, I examine the ways people in nonmonogamous relationships interact with the world: coming out (or not), finding community, and creating support networks. Chapter 17 is concerned with the unique issues people in open relationships face when raising children. Information about safer sex and sexual health is discussed in Chapter 18, and Chapter 19 deals with legal and practical issues.

In Chapter 20, I look toward the future of relationships and share words of advice from my interviewees. At the end of the book are some useful appendixes, including the endnotes, detailed information and statistics about my research subjects, and a Resource Guide. The Resource Guide includes recommended books as well as one of the most comprehensive compilations of national and local organizations, publications, events, websites, and online communities.

I chose the title *Opening Up* because I like all that it implies about people in open relationships. They're open to suggestion. Open to interpretation. Open to possibilities. Their desires aren't guarded, but out in the open. These people make room in their beds, lives, and hearts for other people. To those who explore the possibilities beyond monogamy, opening up is about expanding and evolving. Everyone I interviewed opened up to me. Some of them were content and settled, while others were at a crossroads in their relationship, with uncertainty ahead of them. They all shared their worries, their fears, their hopes, and their dreams. Their stories touched my life in innumerable ways, and I hope they touch yours on your journey toward opening up.

Tristan Taormino

Chapter 1

Pilots, Parties, and Polyamory: A Brief History

THE PRACTICE OF conducting consensual multiple sex and love relationships simultaneously is not new. As long as people have been in relationships, there have been open relationships. From swinging and open marriage to gay and lesbian sex spaces and communes, a look at models from recent history provides a context for today's open relationships.

Swinging

In the United States, swinging was the first organized form of modern nonmonogamy for heterosexual and bisexual people. Swinging began as a hidden subculture, so its history is hard to track, but there is speculation about its beginnings. Organized parties where people had sex with one another date from the 1930s and 1940s in Hollywood. One theory is that swinging began among Air Force fighter pilots and their wives during World War II. Pilots moved their wives close to base, where a tight-knit community of pilots and wives formed. Because so many pilots died in combat, it was understood that surviving pilots would care for widows as they would their own wives. This practice supposedly continued through the Korean War. A slightly different theory is that swinging began on military bases in California in the 1950s. Neither theory has been well documented or verified. We do know that in the late 1950s the media reported on a new phenomenon in the suburbs called "wife swapping." There is also much folklore about "key parties" in the sixties and seventies—where the husbands placed their keys in a bowl and each wife picked a set and had sex with whomever they belonged to. Another theory is that swinging began among hippies and nudists, and some people point to the Sexual Freedom League, a liberal activist group founded in 1960s Berkeley which held orgy parties.[1]

By the mid- to late sixties, swinger groups formed and swing parties moved out of the underground, becoming popular among mainly white, affluent heterosexual couples who lived in the suburbs, and the parties were no longer so secretive that they couldn't be found. For their 1964 book *Swap Clubs*,[2] William and Jerrye Breedlove talked to 800 people who belonged to swinger groups in more than 25 cities in nearly every region of the United States. The Breedloves' study was part of a surge of sociological research on swingers in the late sixties and seventies. Academics' fascination with swinging resulted in dozens of journal articles and books such as *Open Marriage*, by Nena and George O'Neill, *Group Marriage*, by Larry and Joan Constantine, *Beyond Monogamy*, edited by James R. Smith and Lynn G. Smith, and Ronald Mazur's *The New Intimacy: Open-Ended Marriage and Alternative Lifestyles*. Swingers themselves chimed in, writing several self-help-style handbooks, including *Together Sex* and *The Civilized Couple's Guide to Extramarital Adventure*.

In 1969, Robert and Geri McGinley founded a weekly social group for swingers that eventually became the Lifestyles Organization, one of the oldest and largest swinger organizations in the country. The organization produced the first Lifestyles Convention in 1973, and by the 1980s Lifestyles Conventions were attracting over 1,000 couples.

In the late 1970s, Robert McGinley created the North American Swing Club Association (NASCA), a trade organization for swing clubs; today hundreds of swinger-related businesses belong to NASCA, which has become an international organization.[3]

Since the 1960s, various researchers have estimated the number of people who swing at between 1 and 8 million. In the late 1990s, McGinley estimated that there were about 3 million swingers in the US based on the number of clubs, roster of club memberships, attendance at parties, and samples of private parties in selected cities.[4] Today, swingers are a large, organized subculture with their own magazines, websites, clubs, parties, and conventions. They routinely "take over" entire hotels and resorts for their events.

Utopian Swingers

Among academics who wrote about swingers in the late sixties and seventies, sociologist Carolyn Symonds was the first to classify swingers as either "recreational" or "utopian." She described recreational swingers as "persons who use swinging as a form of recreation... It might fill needs for socializing, exercise, or perhaps sexual variety or conquest." She identified utopian swingers as a much smaller group of "philosophical utopians who dream of forming a community and living all aspects of their lives in that environment. They want to share not only sex with their fellow communitarians but also provision for food and shelter, childrearing, education, and other areas of living."[5] Other researchers of that period went on to adopt, critique, and reject the terms. What is most useful about Symonds's classification is that she identified a small subset of people who differed from the majority, one that was more politicized and not threatened by the development of additional love relationships. The utopian swinger sounds very much like an early prototype of the polyamorous person.

Open Marriage

In 1972, when most discussions about nonmonogamy concerned swinging, Nena and George O'Neill proposed a new relationship model that could include nonmonogamy. Their book *Open Marriage: A New Life Style for Couples*, based on interviews they conducted as well as their own personal philosophies, sold over 1.5 million copies. The O'Neills summarized their vision for an open marriage:

> Open marriage thus can be defined as a relationship in which the partners are committed to their own and to each other's growth. It is an honest and open relationship of intimacy and self-disclosure based on the equal freedom and identity of both partners. Supportive caring and increasing security in individual identities make possible the sharing of self-growth with a meaningful other who encourages and anticipates his own and his mate's growth. It is a relationship that is flexible enough to allow for change and that is constantly being renegotiated in the light of changing needs, consensus in decision-making, acceptance and encouragement of individual growth, and openness to new possibilities for growth.[6]

Employing some of the trends of the self-help movement of the time, the O'Neills put forth a new concept of marriage where spouses rejected rigid roles, emphasized open and honest communication, and pursued freedom. They envisioned open marriage as a tool for personal growth (as evidenced by their use of the word *growth* five times in the brief description above). After the book was published, the O'Neills attempted to deemphasize the issue of sexual nonmonogamy, yet the term *open marriage* became synonymous with a sexually open marriage.

Multilateral Marriage

In 1973, husband and wife Larry and Joan Constantine coined the term *multilateral marriage* in their groundbreaking book *Group Marriage: A Study of Contemporary Multilateral Marriage*. Spurred by their own experience and interest in group marriage, the Constantines decided to begin a study of people in group marriages. Without conventional credentials—they were not sociologists or therapists, though Larry Constantine was studying for a Certificate in Family Therapy at the Boston Family Institute—they set out to locate people living in group marriages and conduct detailed interviews with them by mail and in person. They found subjects through underground networks, hard-to-find support groups, and word of mouth, and as their study got under way, subjects began contacting them. For three years, they mailed interviews to people and traveled around the country to interview them in person, driving 32,000 miles in their Volkswagen Squareback with a trailer in tow. In total, there were 104 participants in the study.

The Constantines defined multilateral marriage as a relationship that "consists of three or more partners, each of whom considers himself/herself to be married," intending to distinguish it from the term *group marriage*, which referred to a four-person marriage between two men and two women.[7] They were among the first (if not the first) to use the terms *cowife* and *cohusband* to describe the relationships between partners within a multilateral marriage. They studied a fairly diverse group of people (though gays and lesbians are absent from their research—it was the 70s, and finding straight groups proved difficult enough) and made astute observations about them. Multilateral marriage was the prototype of modern polyfidelity, a style of polyamory.

Gay Bathhouses and Sex Clubs

Swinging, open marriage, and multilateral marriage were the first forms of organized, documented nonmonogamy for heterosexuals. Public, recreational, and multipartner sex among gay men has been traced back to before swinging. Gay historian Allan Bérubé writes, "Before there were any openly gay or lesbian leaders, political clubs, books, films, newspapers, businesses, neighborhoods, churches, or legally recognized gay rights, several generations of pioneers spontaneously created gay bathhouses."[8] In the late 19th and early 20th century, in addition to places like parks, YMCAs, and public restrooms, Turkish baths and other public baths in major cities became sites where men had sex with other men. From the 1920s to the 1950s, certain bathhouses developed a strong gay following and became relatively safe spaces where men could meet, socialize, and have anonymous, casual, or no-strings-attached sex with other men, often in private cubbies or rooms. During the 1950s, the first bathhouses openly marketed to a gay clientele opened in San Francisco and New York, marking the first time public gay male sex was organized and community-based. In the 1960s, in response to the "free love" movement of the era, bathhouses began installing orgy rooms for group sex.[9] By the seventies, gay male sex, fisting, and S/M clubs were being founded in San Francisco, New York, and other cities.

When gay male culture was underground and criminalized, bathhouses and bars were among the few places for men to meet each other. Yet after being gay became more accepted and a visible gay community emerged, bathhouses remained—and to this day still remain—an important, thriving part of gay male culture. Bathhouses exist all over the country and are frequented by single men, partnered men, and couples who go together. The presence of bathhouses and their longevity in gay culture represents how casual sex and nonmonogamy (both consensual and not) have been part of gay communities.

In her essay about the infamous San Francisco fisting and S/M club the Catacombs, Gayle Rubin refers to the underlying relationships formed through public sex spaces: "Places devoted to sex are usually depicted as harsh, alienated, scary environments, where people have only the most utilitarian and exploitative relationships. The Catacombs could not have been more different… It was a sexually organized environment where people treated each other with mutual respect, and where they were lovingly sexual without being in holy wedlock."[10] Jack Fritscher echoes Rubin's sentiments in his recollection of some of the nontraditional relationships that came out of the Catacombs:

> I think particularly of Cynthia Slater, the founder of the Janus Society, with whom I played Top many times at the Catacombs—which was interesting because outside the Catacombs, Cynthia was herself conducting a sexual affair with my brother (yes, my real actual straight brother), just as she was being photographed by my bicoastal lover, Robert Mapplethorpe, to whom I introduced her. Cynthia liked my brother, because he was straight and he could fuck her while I could Top her in S/M, so she got two very similar guys in, like, one huge experience. Oh, fuck it: she, he, and I—it was soooo 70s! So "Twosies beats onesies, but nothing beats threes" from *Cabaret*.[11]

In addition to public and multipartner sex, other kinds of nonmonogamy among gay men are quite common. As the community and culture evolved, gay men, especially those interested in S/M and public sex, were already renegades of mainstream society, and it seems only logical that they would forge new relationship styles rather than sticking to straight, monogamous ones.

Lesbian Collectives and Sex Wars

During the women's movement of the 1970s, all-women (and specifically all-lesbian) cooperative living situations were born. Women sought to create lives free of sexism and other forms of oppression in alternative utopias where they shared childrearing duties, living space, and resources. Part of the communal philosophy was to envision and bring to life nonpatriarchal models, including those for sex and relationships. In her account of living in one such collective in Oregon, Thyme S. Siegel writes about these emerging villages: "Emerald City's Matriarchal Village was one place among many, on country land and in college towns of the 1970s, where lesbian villages emerged. Most of these villages were characterized by various sorts of 'nonmonogamy,' harmonious and not."[12]

In the late seventies and eighties, as gay male sex and S/M clubs emerged in urban areas, women were allowed into these clubs in rare cases (as at the Catacombs in San Francisco). Lesbian and bisexual women began to "borrow" these spaces for their own parties, and eventually lesbian sex and S/M events happened on a regular basis both at clubs and private parties; this created a physical space for communities to begin to coalesce—communities of women interested in power play, public and multipartner sex, and alternative relationship structures. The lesbian sex magazine *On Our Backs* debuted in 1984; in addition to explicit photography, one issue contained an essay on group sex by then editor Susie Bright. During the sex wars of the 1980s, while anti-S/M lesbian feminists and lesbian feminist sex radicals found themselves on opposites sides of arguments about sex, porn, and sadomasochism, some of them did agree on one thing: monogamy should not be assumed or necessarily embraced.

The 1990s and early 2000s brought a surge of writing by queer women about nontraditional sexuality and relationships, including *Lesbian Polyfidelity*, by Celeste West; *The Lesbian Polyamory Reader*, edited by Marcia Munson and Judith P. Stelboum; writing by Pat Califia, Susie Bright, Shar Rednour, and Carol Queen; essays in *Bi Any Other Name* and *Coming to Power: A Leatherdyke Reader*; as well as dozens of erotica anthologies. In her 1996 book *Lesbian Polyfidelity*, Celeste West reported that 20 percent of her lesbian respondents were polyamorous.

Polyamory

Some sources state that the word *polyamory* may have roots as far back as the 1960s. The concept and basic principles of consensual, responsible nonmonogamy emerged before the term *polyamory* was actually coined. As swinger and gay and lesbian communities thrived in California in the seventies, a different form of nonmonogamy emerged in San Francisco: utopian communes. One of the best known is the Kerista Commune (also known as Kerista Village), which began to take shape amid the free love and hippie movements of the era. The Kerista Commune was a community founded in the early to mid-seventies by Jud Presmont. Keristans coined the term *polyfidelity* (faithful to many partners) to describe this new relationship form in which each woman in the group had a sexual and love relationship with each man, complete with a "balanced rotational sleeping schedule" that determined who slept with whom; no one had sex or relationships outside the group. The number of Kerista members varied from about eight to as many as 30, and each member agreed to a social contract that included hundreds of points. They eventually formed a profitable computer business together. At its height, Kerista was a model of a new consensual, conscious, multipartner relationship style. Kerista officially disbanded in 1991.[13]

In 1984, Ryam Nearing published the first issue of *Loving More*, a newsletter dedicated to the exploration of consensual multiple loving relationships; in the eighties, Nearing also began organizing conferences for people who wore exploring those relationships. At the time, the articles that appeared in *Loving More* used terms like *polyfidelity*, *open relationships*, and *intimate networks*, but many of the ideas discussed were precursors to polyamory. In 1991, *Loving More* became a magazine cofounded by Nearing and Deborah Taj Anapol.[14]

People began identifying themselves as polyamorous, and the concept of polyamorous relationships and communities first emerged, in the 1990s. The term *polyamory* has been attributed to two sources. In a 1990 article titled "A Bouquet of Lovers: Strategies for Responsible Open Relationships," Morning Glory Zell-Ravenheart used the term *poly-amorous* to describe a lifestyle of multiple partners, though she uses *polygamy* (not *polyamory*) as the noun. In 1992, Jennifer Wesp created the Usenet newsgroup alt.polyamory.[15]

The nineties produced several important contributions to defining and understanding polyamory. Five books on the subject were published, including Ryam Nearing's *Loving More: The Polyfidelity Primer* and Deborah Taj Anapol's *Love Without Limits*. *The Ethical Slut: A Guide to Infinite Sexual Possibilities*, by Dossie Easton and Catherine A. Liszt (a pseudonym for Janet Hardy), is arguably the most influential one, considered by many to be the bible of polyamory. It was published in 1997, has been cited in hundreds of other works on polyamory, and, incidentally, was mentioned by at least 80 percent of my interviewees in the course of discussing how they first came to learn about polyamory. In the next decade, as the Internet grew in popularity, poly people found many ways to connect with one another online.

Today, there are hundreds, maybe thousands, of local and national organizations, support groups, Listservs, and online communities, plus conferences, events, and websites dedicated to polyamory. (See the Resource Guide.) There has not been enough research on polyamorous people to produce many meaningful statistics about the number of people currently or formerly in some kind of consensual nonmonogamous relationship. In their 1983 study, Philip Blumstein and Pepper

Schwartz reported that of 3,574 couples in their sample, 15 percent of married couples had "an understanding that allows nonmonogamy under some circumstances." Those percentages were higher among cohabiting couples (28 percent), lesbian couples (29 percent), and gay male couples (65 percent).[16] The Janus Report sampled 1,800 people (1993), 21 percent of whom said they participated in open marriage.[17] In a much smaller 2004 study of 217 bisexual people, E. H. Page found that 33 percent were involved in a polyamorous relationship and 54 percent considered polyamory ideal.[18] In 2007, when Oprah.com conducted a survey of over 14,000 people, 21 percent said they were in an open marriage.[19]

Chapter 2

Myths about Nonmonogamy

FROM RELIGION AND RHETORIC to pundits and punch lines, misconceptions about nonmonogamy are everywhere in our society, making them hard to escape and easy to internalize. It is important to expose and correct misinformed, negative mythology to gain a better understanding of what nonmonogamy really is and what it's not before you can fairly consider all your relationship options. Exposing the bias behind the myths and revealing the facts can also help you respond to criticism from others.

Human beings were meant to be monogamous; like other animals, it's how we bond and mate.

In their book *The Myth of Monogamy: Fidelity and Infidelity in Animals and People,* David P. Barash and Judith Eve Lipton argue just the opposite: "In attempting to maintain a social and sexual bond consisting exclusively of one man and one woman, aspiring monogamists are going against some of the deepest-seated evolutionary inclinations with which biology has endowed most creatures, *Homo sapiens* included."[1] It's well documented that most animal species are actually not monogamous. Out of

4,000 species, only a few dozen choose one mate, have sex with only that mate, and stay with that mate until one or both die(s).[2]

Open relationships are unnatural, abnormal, and immoral.

This myth is based on the notion that monogamy is natural, normal, and moral, and any relationship style that isn't monogamous is wrong. As a society, we establish certain norms that change over time. These norms are reinforced by institutions, including religion, government, and the media. Our "nature" to be nonmonogamous has been documented by science (see previous myth). What is normal is always open to debate. As for what is moral, unfortunately, religious conservatives have a stranglehold on morality in this country. Our morality is supposed to guide us to determine what's right and wrong. In my book, what's right is following your heart and creating honest, ethical relationships that work for you.

Polyamory is what Mormons practice.

Polygamy, a term used by academics, anthropologists, and researchers primarily for classification purposes, is the practice of one person having multiple spouses or partners. It exists in three forms: polygyny, polyandry, and group marriage. *Polygyny* is the practice of one man having several wives or female partners; *polyandry* is the practice of one woman having multiple husbands or male partners; *group marriage* is a combination of polygyny and polyandry.

In the United States, polygamy is most closely associated with Mormonism. Beginning in the 1830s, the founder of The Church of Jesus Christ of Latter-day Saints, Joseph Smith, preached and practiced plural marriage as an integral part of the Mormon faith. Smith's successor Brigham Young continued to promote plural marriage. The Church of Jesus Christ of Latter-day Saints officially outlawed polygamy in 1890. Today, according to the leadership of the church, only certain fundamentalist sects of Mormonism teach polygamy as central to the religion and continue to practice it. What they practice is actually polygyny (one man with multiple wives), though it is most often referred to as polygamy or plural marriage. According to an informal survey reported in the *Salt Lake Tribune*, there are 37,000 Mormon fundamentalists in the United States, and about half live in polygamous relationships.[3]

The most controversial issue associated with the practice of polygamy by Mormon fundamentalists is the issue of consent. Many Mormon ex-polygamists have made claims of coercion, kidnapping, brainwashing, incest, and abuse, especially of young women who are married to much older men without their consent. There are non-Mormons who practice consensual multipartner relationships that fit the literal definition of polygamy; however, they usually call themselves *polyamorous* or *polyfidelitous*.

People in open relationships have psychological problems.

Research based on standard psychological testing has shown that people in nonmonogamous relationships are no more or less dysfunctional, narcissistic, neurotic, pathological, psychotic, or generally fucked up than people in monogamous relationships.[4] This doesn't mean people in open relationships are all well-adjusted and psychologically healthy. It just means that there's no difference between monogamous and non-monogamous people when it comes this stuff. However, one study showed that an individual in an open relationship tends to be "individualistic, an academic achiever, creative, nonconforming, stimulated by complexity and chaos, inventive, relatively unconventional and indifferent to what others said, concerned about his/her own personal values and ethical systems, and willing to take risks to explore possibilities."[5] Because open relationships require well-developed relationship skills, people in them tend to have more self-awareness, better communication skills, and a better sense of self.

People in open relationships have intimacy issues and trouble with commitment.

The assumption underlying this myth is that true intimacy can only be achieved between two people in a monogamous relationship. In other words, if you are emotionally and physically intimate with more than one person, it somehow "dilutes" the intimacy of each relationship. This is based on the notion that love is a quantifiable thing: If you have 100 pounds of love, you can give 100 pounds to your partner, but if you have multiple partners, you have to split the 100 pounds between them. Intimacy is about being willing to be open, honest, and vulnerable with your partner and bonding on a deep level. Monogamy does not automatically foster intimacy in a relationship, any more than non-monogamy fosters a lack of intimacy. Furthermore, nonmonogamous relationships often involve the same level of commitment as monogamous ones. People in nonmonogamous relationships are not avoiding intimacy or commitment, they are cultivating a relationship style that meets their needs and works for them.

If you're nonmonogamous, it's because you are confused and indecisive.

This myth goes along with the previous one, the idea that nonmonogamous people cannot commit to one person or choose between them. It's quite the opposite: most nonmonogamous people are very clear about why they choose nonmonogamy and what they want and need out of their relationships. And it's not that they *can't* choose between partners, it's that they don't want to and believe strongly that they don't have to.

Polyamory is just a fancy term for promiscuity.

While a polyamorous person may have several lovers, polyamory is not simply all about sex. Polyamorous relationships may encompass friendship, companionship, support, camaraderie, love, intimacy, connection, commitment. All that said, having an active sex life with more than one person isn't a bad thing.

Nonmonogamy is physically dangerous; you're more likely to get diseases because you have multiple partners.

Having multiple sexual partners at the same time does not automatically put you at greater risk for sexually transmitted infections (STIs). Having unprotected sex with an individual infected with an STI or an individual whose STI status you do not know puts you at greater risk for contracting an STI. There is no evidence that nonmonogamous people have a higher rate of STIs than monogamous people. Furthermore, every person I interviewed cited safer sex as one of the main rules of their open relationships.

Nonmonogamy is no different from cheating.

Cheating involves lying, deception, and breaking a commitment previously made. For nonmonogamy to be successful, everyone must tell the truth and respect the rules agreed upon. Consensual nonmonogamy means that all parties involved have agreed to the arrangement.

Polyamory is an unhealthy environment in which to raise kids.

Children need parents and other adults in their lives who are committed to raising them with love, support, respect, and understanding. Although conservatives want us to believe that the heterosexual nuclear family is the best environment in which to raise children, that family unit has been shown over and over to be as dysfunctional as any other type of family—if not more so. Today, plenty of children are raised by so-called nontraditional families consisting of one mother, two mothers, one father, two fathers, two divorced parents, one or more stepparents, a grandparent, or some combination thereof. The important thing is for children to have stability and for parents to be honest with them about their relationships.

Chapter 3

Is an Open Relationship for You?

FROM SEXUAL VARIETY AND FANTASY to personal growth and fulfillment, there are many different reasons why people choose non-monogamy. Before I outline some of the popular motivations, I'll caution you against some potentially problematic ones. If you are considering expanding your monogamous relationship to a nonmonogamous one, don't do so out of discontent or dissatisfaction with your current relationship, believing that bringing other people into the mix will fix it. This is a surefire path to disaster—opening up the relationship will only highlight its problems. Don't attempt an open relationship because you think it's the cool, hip thing to do or because everyone around you is in one. Also, you should not feel pressured or coerced by your partner to explore nonmonogamy. You both must be on the same page if it's going to have a chance of working.

Self-evaluation

If you are considering an open relationship, first evaluate yourself thoroughly and honestly to determine whether venturing beyond monogamy is right for you. Here are some questions for you to contemplate, write about in a journal, or talk about with a friend, partner, or therapist:

What are your beliefs about monogamy?
- If you've been in monogamous relationships before, how did you feel in those relationships, and how did they work or not work for you?
- Do you believe that someone can love/be in love with more than one person at a time?
- What role does sex play in your relationships? How important is it to you? What does it mean to you?
- Can you have sex without an emotional attachment? How are sex and love related or not related?
- Have you ever had a "fuck buddy" or "friend with benefits"? What worked and didn't work about the relationship?

If you are currently in a relationship:
- What is the state of the relationship? Does it feel stable and secure?
- What are your most common conflicts with your partner?
- Do both partners want to explore a different structure?
- Do you have sexual needs, desires, and fantasies that aren't being fulfilled?

Imagine your partner having sex with another person. It's important to be brutally honest, not censor yourself, and really let yourself feel what that would be like.
- What feelings does that bring up?
- What would be your worst fear?
- What would the best-case scenario for this situation look like?
- What would be an absolute deal breaker?

Imagine your partner having a relationship with another person. It's important to be brutally honest, not censor yourself, and really let yourself feel what that would be like.

- What feelings does that bring up?
- What would be your worst fear?
- What would the best-case scenario for this situation look like?
- What would be an absolute deal breaker?

How do you handle feelings?

- Do you consider yourself a jealous person? How do you deal with intense feelings like anger, jealousy, and resentment?
- Are you able to determine what your boundaries are and communicate them to others?
- When something is bothering you, do you more often keep it to yourself or share it?
- Do you have the ability to communicate openly and honestly, even about difficult issues?
- When conflict arises, how do you usually handle it?

How available are you?

- Do you have the time to nurture and grow more than one love relationship?
- Do you have the energy to devote to several different people and juggle multiple lovers?
- Do you have access to potential partners who have nonmonogamy experience and strong relationship skills?
- Do you have the self-knowledge and communication skills to be in an open relationship?

Why People Choose Open Relationships

If you've never been in an open relationship of any kind, you may be wondering why people choose them and what they get out of them.

People choose to create nonmonogamous relationships for many different reasons, and I will explore some of the most common in this chapter. One or more of the following may ring true for you or echo your own experience.

Sexual and Fantasy Fulfillment

For those who have a primary partner and choose to explore only sex (no emotional attachment or relationships) with other people, erotic desire is the driving force. Maybe you've always had fantasies about sex with someone other than your current partner, bringing a third person into the bedroom, or hooking up at a party while others watched. Many long-term couples find that having additional sexual partners keeps their relationship fresh, breaks up monotony and routine, adds excitement to their sex life, and brings them closer to each other.

How can sex with someone else increase the intimacy between primary partners? For some people, sharing their fantasies with each other—even if those fantasies are about other people—is an important step toward building closeness. Eli likes to explore with other people different kinds of sex that his partner doesn't enjoy; he says, "It enables me to show different aspects of my sexuality to those who appreciate them most." When couples explore a fantasy together, it can be a special, exciting, bonding event; just as some couples go mountain-climbing or skydiving together, others go on sexual adventures. You can talk about your experiences afterward, and your different perspectives may give you new insight into each other's sexuality.

> *In general, after a night of [playing with others], we are very hot for each other, have the most amazing sex, and have the strongest feelings of confidence in our own relationship. —Jack*

Rejection of Monogamy

Many people say that their discovery of nonmonogamy resulted from their dissatisfaction with monogamy: the monogamous relationships they've had just didn't seem like a good fit for them. Some feel that the structure and expectations of monogamy are confining, stifling, and unnatural and that they simply aren't "wired" for monogamy. From the time they began dating and having relationships, they've always preferred several partners to just one, and they enjoy exploring different kinds of relationships and dynamics with different people. In an interview about the study she conducted on brain activity of people in love, Helen Fisher, author of *Why We Love: The Nature and Chemistry of Romantic Love*, says:

> I have a theory that we've evolved three distinctly different brain systems for mating and reproduction. The sex drive being one, that craving for sexual gratification. The second is romantic love, that obsession, the craving, the ecstasy, the focused attention, the motivation to win a particular mating partner; that early, intense romantic love. And the third brain system is attachment, that sense of calm and security that you can feel with a long-term partner.
>
> What I find most remarkable about these three drives...is that they're often unconnected. You can feel a powerful sense of attachment to a long-term partner while you feel intense romantic love for somebody else, while you feel this sex drive for a whole range of people.[1]

Fisher's conclusions support the folks who simply cannot imagine themselves in any kind of relationship other than an open one, like Shari, who says, "I've never had a monogamous fantasy in my life...I just never, ever, dreamt of 'him.' I always dreamt of 'them,' from the earliest days of my sexual fantasizing. My sexuality is very fluid and wide-ranging."

Freedom and Openness

Freedom is one of the major draws of an open relationship. Many who choose nonmonogamy appreciate the freedom they have to acknowledge their attraction to multiple people—whether they act on those feelings or not.

According to societal expectations, you might be single or dating, but the inherent assumption is you're actively looking for "the one" and want to "settle down." If you're living with someone, engaged, or married, you're assumed to be monogamous. Within a committed relationship, the expectations get even more specific. Open relationships can give you the freedom to create unique relationships, explore yourself and your sexuality, and challenge society's expectations.

> *Putting limits on love is like putting a leash on me. Even if it isn't tight around my neck, knowing it's there is enough... I like being with my partners because I want to, not because I have to.* —Juan

Many people find themselves in relationships that just don't fit the limited categories or definitions of mainstream society. Rather than trying to cram a nontraditional relationship into the framework of a traditional one, nonmonogamous people want to redefine relationships, commitment, fidelity, partnership—and even marriage—on their terms. Arielle says, "Polyamory gives me the opportunity to have relationships up and down the spectrum and appreciate them for what they are."

Sexual and Emotional Diversity

Each person's sexuality is incredibly specific and unique. When you meet a partner with whom you are sexually compatible, many of your tastes and desires overlap. But that doesn't mean that everything is a perfect match. When a sexual difference emerges, you could reject the partner as not a perfect match and move on, or let your desire go unfulfilled. Some people take a different route: they choose to explore with other partners the sexual needs and wants that don't "fit" in their committed relationship with one partner. The notion of an open relationship often comes up when a significant difference between partners emerges and must be addressed—for example, when she discovers her bisexuality, or he discovers his desire to crossdress, and their partner cannot or will not fulfill that particular sexual need.

It's a common scenario for one partner to be kinky and the other one not. Rather than ask one partner to deny his or her desire for dominance and submission, or bondage, or different forms of sensation play, the couple agrees to open the relationship to accommodate the attraction to kink. (In this discussion I use the term *kink* interchangeably with *BDSM*, an umbrella term that includes a wide range of intimate activities—physical, sexual, psychological, spiritual, or a combination—that usually involve an exchange of power. BD stands for bondage and discipline; D/s for dominance/submission; S/M for sadism/masochism, or sadomasochism.)

Dani, who had been married for 10 years, saw a special on HBO about BDSM one day. She got really excited and wanted to explore it. Her husband agreed to give it a try, but he just didn't like it. As Dani put it, "It was hard at first, but as soon as he came to an understanding of what I needed, and that he either couldn't or didn't want to give it, then he said, 'You need to find it someplace else.'"

Even if both partners identify as kinky, many of their specific likes may not overlap. For example, one woman identifies as a Top (the doer, the one who runs the scene); her partner is a bottom who loves to be flogged and spanked, but really isn't into psychological play—they tried it a few times together and it just didn't work. Because they have an open relationship, they are free to explore activities their partner doesn't enjoy. I've also witnessed relationships begin with one dynamic, for example, Daddy/boy, only to change when the boy figures out one day that he's more of a Dominant (the person who is in control or wields authority over the submissive). The couple can transition into a relationship without a Dominant/submissive dynamic, and each can find other people to play with. This allows them to keep a valued relationship intact while also recognizing that a significant change has occurred and needs to be addressed. Because our desires are often complex, erotic differences can be much more subtle than simply bisexual/straight or kinky/nonkinky.

> *Since I am a bisexual switch with a vanilla streak married to a nonswitching Dom, if we weren't open sexually we couldn't be together, no matter how deep our love for each other. Having outside partners to fill in the gaps in our compatibility prevents resentment and ill will; this way, no one is viewed as deficient in any way, or seen as inadequate.* —Shari

Perhaps you and your partner have not identified a specific difference or incompatibility, but you've always had the desire for emotional and erotic diversity with multiple partners. Society would have us believe that one person should fulfill all of our needs and desires: physical, emotional, financial, sexual, spiritual, and all the rest. This is the myth of finding "the One": the one partner you're "meant" to be with, your soul mate, your Prince Charming, the girl of your dreams. Nonmonogamous folks reject this myth and acknowledge that no one person can be, or should be expected to be, everything for another. People in open relationships enjoy exploring different dynamics with different people—sexual, emotional, psychological, and spiritual. Nonmonogamy gives them the opportunity to create unique relationships that nourish and support each other.

> *I am someone's soul mate, someone's youth, someone's slut, someone's girlfriend. Sometimes I am all of those at once. My partners inspire me to love, take care of me, call me their slut, and take me out for sushi. It's good to have all those qualities, and rare to find them in one person.* —Hannah

Polyamory helps me not feel frustrated or resentful towards one partner if they aren't everything to me. —Callie

Many people in monogamous relationships deal with cheating all the time: the fear of cheating, the suspicion of cheating, the discovery of cheating, the aftermath of cheating. Nonmonogamous folks recognize that during a lifetime you can and will be attracted to other people even if you are in a wonderful, fulfilling relationship; they make room in their relationship for these attractions rather than allow them to cause anxiety, jealousy, and unreasonable expectations.

I get to live in the realness of knowing that my partner and I have desires for others and we are able to negotiate and explore them with respect to each other as primaries. —Khane

Mixed-Orientation Marriages

It is estimated that nationwide about 2 million gay men and lesbians currently have or formerly had a straight spouse.[2] Amity Pierce Buxton, author of *The Other Side of the Closet: The Coming-Out Crisis for Straight Spouses and Families*, has interviewed over 9,000 gay and straight spouses since the mid-80s. Buxton says that when one partner in a marriage comes out as gay, lesbian, or bisexual, about a third of the couples break up right away, a third break up after about two years, and a third stay married indefinitely.[3] We don't know a whole lot about that last third—the more than 30 percent of mixed-orientation marriages that remain intact. From the research I've read, many of them are negotiating open relationships, but few consider themselves polyamorous or identify with or seek out a nonmonogamous community. As a result, they are left out of significant discussions about nonmonogamy.

Research and writing on this topic (including Buxton's) makes a point of distinguishing between partners who come out as gay or lesbian and partners who come out as bisexual. Those are individual identity choices; I am less concerned with how a person identifies and more interested in the relationship between the straight spouse and the nonstraight spouse, because that ultimately determines what style of open relationship will work for them. Some couples remain primary partners and continue to have a sexual relationship, while others end the sexual element of their partnership. In one of Buxton's studies, the straight husband of a bisexual woman wrote: "I compare my wife and me to a glove with fingers that fit absolutely perfect. It's the thumb that is just wrong. The more we struggle to make the thumb fit, the worse off we make the fingers. If we free ourselves to adjust the gloves for our thumbs, then the fingers return to their old wonderful fit."[4]

One of the most difficult issues facing mixed-orientation marriages is that they began as one thing—heterosexual marriage—and must transform into something radically different—an open relationship with no script, no plan, and usually no support, understanding, or acceptance from society. Unlike unmarried couples and couples with the same orientation, these couples don't sit down one day to negotiate an open marriage in the absence of a serious event: the coming out of one spouse prompts the change, and they are restructuring their relationship essentially to keep it from ending.

Personal and Spiritual Growth

Some folks consciously choose open relationships as a path for personal growth and the growth of their relationships. They want to be challenged by their relationships. They want to push themselves to confront feelings like jealousy, possessiveness, or attachment, and work through these emotions to gain greater self-awareness. They want to learn and change through their relationships.

> I am a very independent, autonomous, adventurous person. I start
> to feel suffocated and antsy when my life feels too domestic and
> mundane. Multiple relationships force me to stay in the moment

*and on my toes emotionally, to communicate better, and to face
fear on a weekly basis.* —Elizabeth

Similarly, some polyamorous people see their relationship style as a
fundamental part of their spirituality. They believe that opening oneself
up to multiple relationships is part of their spiritual identity and practice.
Kathleen, who calls herself "technically Pagan with some Buddhist and
Gnostic Christian," says, "Part of my job on the planet is to express and
experience love. We traditionally have a very narrow view of how you
should do that. I don't think there's necessarily a 'one soul mate.' I think
if there's a loving god out there, why would he limit us to only one?"

Some of My Best Friends Are Monogamous

After some careful self-reflection, you may decide that monogamy is
your preferred relationship style. Great! A disturbing trend among some
nonmonogamous people is to turn their noses up at those who choose
monogamy, casting them as naïve, boring, brainwashed, unfulfilled, and
unevolved—as if everyone in an open relationship is worldly, exciting,
freethinking, fulfilled, and evolved simply by being nonmonogamous!
The truth is, many people do not consciously choose monogamy; society chooses it for them, and it becomes the default. They're not aware
that other options exist or could actually work. Many people don't give
any other option a second thought, and their relationships suffer as a
result. But I also know plenty of folks who've done a great deal of exper-
imenting, soul-searching, and self-analysis and come to the conclusion
that monogamy is the relationship style that works best for them. This
book is not about valuing one relationship choice over another. My mis-
sion in sex and relationship education has always been to empower
people to explore all their options, discover what works best for them,
and go out and get it.

There is no one "right" reason for deciding to create an open relationship; however, there is a common theme in what inspires people to step outside monogamy: making a conscious, thoughtful choice to do what works best for them, even if what works best goes against society's norms. If you decide that nonmonogamy is worth looking into, the next step is to figure out what your version of nonmonogamy looks like, then try it. Various forms of nonmonogamy *could* work for anyone, in theory. The true test is to jump in with both feet and see if it works for you in practice.

EXERCISE

Benefits and Challenges

Creating a list of pros and cons may be helpful as you assess whether an open relationship is right for you. I like to think of the pros and cons as benefits and challenges. Here are some to get you started.

Benefits:

- Avoid feeling stifled, limited, confined
- Be free to acknowledge or to act on attractions, desires
- Be free to create relationships that work for you
- Have multiple sexual partners and experiences
- Have multiple relationships
- Get different needs met with different people
- Explore different sexual or relationship dynamics
- No need to end one relationship to start another
- No need to be all things to one partner and vice versa
- Be challenged to learn and grow through relationships
- Live honestly
- Work on self awareness, jealousy, other issues

Challenges:

- More relationships means more work
- Not enough time
- Lacking a sense of relationship security
- Requires solid communication and negotiation skills
- Requires self-reflection and intense honesty
- Must regularly confront feelings of jealousy and insecurity
- Disapproval of friends, family, community, society

Chapter 4

What Makes an Open Relationship Work?

PEOPLE WHO PRACTICE NONMONOGAMY are a truly diverse bunch and they design their relationships in many different ways. Yet, there are some key emotional skills they have in common, qualities that help them to negotiate and nurture their relationships. If you don't have a clear idea of who you are or what you want, or you feel insecure about yourself and your relationship, it will likely be difficult for you to navigate through nonmonogamy. Engaging in self-reflection, processing your feelings with other people, and being willing to deal with conflict are necessary skills to create alternatives to monogamy. As you continue to ponder whether an open relationship is right for you, consider some of the significant elements that help make these relationships work: consent, self-discovery and self-awareness, communication, honesty, boundaries, trust, fidelity, and commitment.

Consent

I begin with consent because it is a foundational element for all relationships and one of the significant qualities that distinguish nonmonogamy from cheating. To ensure a healthy, positive, fulfilling open relationship, everyone involved must be on board. No one should feel pressured, coerced, or otherwise pushed to be in a relationship they don't want to be in. You should not open up a monogamous relationship or begin a non-monogamous one to please someone else, avoid conflict, or give in to a demand, or because you fear the relationship might otherwise end. Do it because you know what you're getting into and you want to get into it.

It would be unwise to agree to nonmonogamy for the following reasons or with these hidden motives:

- You're so in love with the person that while your gut is telling you no, you decide to say yes and will deal with it later.
- You believe your partner likes the idea as an abstract concept, but it won't actually happen.
- You agree to it, but secretly know you'll be "enough" for your partner and she won't ever want anyone else.
- Although your partner has said he is nonmonogamous by nature, you know you can change him.
- You think it's just a phase and she'll get over it.

Be honest with yourself about what the realities of nonmonogamy are to assess whether it's right for you. If you or a partner aren't sure, or need to work out what you need to feel sure, don't rush it. Do some research and weigh your options. Wait until everyone gets to "yes," even if it means waiting longer than you'd like. Be sure to be very clear about what you or your partner are saying "yes" to. Is your partner agreeing to further discussion, a trial run, or additional partners? You want to hear a thoughtful, well-informed "yes" so everyone feels comfortable moving forward.

Self-awareness

A strong sense of self is key in all relationships and it should be a start-ing point for people considering an open relationship. Until you are clear about who you are, what is important to you, and what you need and want, communicating with others can only go so far. Certainly, you don't need to have it *all* figured out before you begin talking. In fact, it often helps people clarify their thoughts and desires by hashing them out with someone else or getting an outsider's opinion. But the more clarity you have about your wishes, your issues, and your goals, the more you bring to the communication process.

Anita Wagner, a polyamory educator and cofounder of the Chesapeake Polyamory Network, likens self-awareness to emotional intelligence, a concept popularized by the book *Emotional Intelligence*, by Daniel Goleman. Anita says:

> What emotional intelligence means for me is understanding my own emotional wiring. For example, someone who has abandonment or serious self-esteem issues needs to be aware of it. They need to know those issues are going to make them especially vulnerable in succeeding in poly relationships. If they're not working on them and getting a pretty big handle on them, the first time their sweetheart goes out to be with someone else, that abandonment button will get pushed big time. It's hard enough for those of us who are okay in those areas... The more emotional intelligence we have, the easier it will be to withstand emotional challenges.[1]

One thing that came through strongly in my interviews is that there aren't a lot of nonmonogamous people wandering through life with their heads down, just following the crowd. The people I talked to are actively engaged in their own personal growth and the growth of their relationships. They expressed a strong interest in knowing themselves (and others) on a deep level. They seek that self-knowledge through a variety of practices, including psychotherapy and counseling, reading, writing, journaling, blogging, attending workshops and peer support groups, meditation, and various spiritual practices. This

isn't to say that all nonmonogamous people have a greater consciousness than others (my interviewees were a self-selected bunch), but by
doing work on themselves, they are better equipped to be in complex
nontraditional relationships.

Society has prescribed certain expectations when it comes to love
and sexual relationships: what a relationship *should* look like, how each
person *should* behave (and these behaviors are usually dictated by traditional gender roles), how long you *should* see each other before becoming
serious, how often you *should* spend time together, how you *should*
express your love and affection for one another. There are rigid ideas
about all these things and more, beginning with the most obvious one:
that a love relationship happens between two (and only two) people
who have sex and an emotional attachment. Within our monogamy-
centered culture, fidelity is defined as sexual and emotional exclusivity
with one person. These values and many others are continually reinforced all around us—through traditional wedding ceremonies, men's
and women's magazines, talk shows, and mainstream books and movies.
I challenge you to throw all of that stuff away and begin from scratch.
It may seem like a daunting project, but until you let go of what you
think you're supposed to believe and how you're supposed to act, you
cannot figure out what encompasses your ideal relationship(s). (See
sidebar for a helpful exercise.)

Communication

Once you've done some self-reflection about where you are coming
from, it's time to open up the discussion. Ask anyone in an open relationship what makes it work, and one word comes up the most often:
communication. Obviously, communication is a critical part of any
kind of relationship, but when it comes to nonmonogamous relationships, good communication is one of the most important skills you can
have. Nonmonogamy is not for the faint of heart or lazy: be prepared

Creating Authentic Relationships

The questions below deal with issues most people take for granted and let society define for them. You can start with a blank canvas and create your own definitions.

- How do you define intimacy and closeness?
- What constitutes a relationship for you?
- Are there different types of relationships you wish you could have?
- How long should a significant relationship last?
- What is sex? Is it intercourse? Is it more specific: penis-in-vagina or penis-in-ass intercourse? What about manual stimulation and penetration, oral sex, sex toys, BDSM play?
- What kinds of things do you consider intimate? Sex, sexual touch, genital contact, a BDSM scene with no sexual aspect?
- Must you live near a partner for a relationship to be important?
- How do you define fidelity?
- What constitutes loving, affectionate, sexual, and romantic behavior? Where do things like flirting, kissing, love letters, gift giving, dating, courting, phone calls, emails, and instant messages fit into your definitions?
- What does commitment mean to you? How do you define a committed relationship?
- What are the most important things you need in a relationship?
- How important is it for you to live with a partner?
- Realistically, how much time and energy do you have to give to a relationship?

to talk things through, listen with compassion, and process your feelings and your partners' feelings. If this sounds tedious or impossible to you, then you might want to reconsider your relationship style, because talking is a fundamental element of making nonmonogamy work. A lot of people I interviewed said that talking about their feelings makes them feel better. Talking about your feelings can reassure you and your partner(s) and help you better understand a situation, which puts you in a better position to resolve a problem, let it go, and move on.

You will have many conversations, each with its own tone, focus, and goals. Here are some examples of moments that are ripe for a conversation:

- Introducing the idea of having an open relationship
- Designing and negotiating the details of your open relationship
- Checking in when something or someone new comes into the picture
- Checking in and debriefing after a party, date, or play session
- Talking it through when one of you is unhappy or experiencing intense feelings
- Dealing with a conflict and working toward a solution
- Redesigning and renegotiating the details of your open relationship

While each of these discussions will proceed differently, there are general guidelines for good communication. All communication should encompass thoughtful self-assessment, honesty, mutual nonjudgmental support, respect, compassionate listening, and a willingness to compromise if necessary. Set aside time to talk, and go into it with the intent that this will not be a short, breezy conversation or a one-shot deal. Communication must be thorough and must be ongoing. Have reasonable expectations: you may not agree with one another right off the bat, and you may not come to a resolution in just one conversation.

Know going into it that talking about relationships, love, sex, and feelings is difficult and emotionally charged for most people.

If one partner is introducing the idea of an open relationship, the initiator should approach the subject gently. Test the water with something general like "Did you hear that Oprah talked about open marriage on her show? What do you think of that?" rather than something confrontational like "I want to open up our marriage and need you to be on board." Give your partner time and space to respond; remember, you may have been thinking about the topic for a year, but this may be the first time it has occurred to him.

If you are the partner receiving the suggestion, keep an open mind. Listen to your partner without criticism or judgment. Resist the impulse to doubt yourself or to buy into the monogamy myth with thoughts like *Why does she want an open relationship? What about me isn't enough?* If you're both interested, keep talking. Do some reading and research. For tips on negotiating your relationship, check out Chapter 11, Designing Your Open Relationship.

If the conversation is about one partner's jealousy or other intense feelings, your first goal should be to listen. Reassure her of your commitment to the relationship. At the moment when a partner is having intense feelings such as hurt, insecurity, jealousy, or betrayal, acknowledge those feelings, validate and respect them, *even if you don't understand them*. Don't try to talk anyone out of how they're feeling with rational arguments; telling them why they shouldn't feel a certain way will get you nowhere. A more objective opinion and reassurances about what's going on from your perspective can come later.

If a conflict has spurred the conversation, the same rule applies: first listen. Practice patience and compassion, and remember that you are on the same team. Don't attempt to defend your position, argue a point, or come to an agreement. Just listen. Remind one another of your love, affection, and respect. Share your side of the situation, remembering to take responsibility for your feelings and your actions.

Tell each other what you need to resolve the problem. Be prepared to compromise if necessary. It may be helpful to read ahead to Chapter 12, Jealousy and Other Intense Feelings, and Chapter 14, Common Challenges and Problems.

Nonviolent Communication

Nonviolent Communication (NVC) is a communication technique created by clinical psychologist Marshall B. Rosenberg and outlined in his book *Nonviolent Communication: A Language of Life*; the concept has since been adapted all over the world. It can be an effective tool for every kind of communication, especially in your relationships. Many of the people I interviewed said they employ the techniques of Nonviolent Communication as they talk about and negotiate their open relationships. Rosenberg has written dozens of books about NVC, as have others; it is a broad topic. The basic concept of NVC is this:

> Most of us have been educated from birth to compete, judge, demand and diagnose—to think and communicate in terms of what is "right" and "wrong" with people. We express our feelings in terms of what another person has "done to us," instead of a feeling independent of another person. We mix up our basic human needs with the strategies we're using to meet those needs (we say "I want you to spend more time with me," instead of "I'm really needing companionship"). And, we ask for what we'd like using demands, the threat of punishment, guilt, or even the promise of rewards.[2]

NVC works by retraining people in how to listen, talk, and express their needs:

> NVC guides us in reframing how we express ourselves and hear others. Instead of being habitual, automatic reactions, our words become conscious responses based firmly on an

awareness of what we are perceiving, feeling, and wanting. We are led to express ourselves with honesty and clarity, while simultaneously paying others a respectful and empathic attention. In any exchange, we come to hear our own deeper needs and those of others. NVC trains us to observe carefully, and to be able to specify behaviors and conditions that are affecting us. We learn to identify and clearly articulate what we are concretely wanting in a given situation.[3]

These are some of the tools of NVC:
- Listening with compassion instead of becoming defensive, attacking, or disconnecting
- Learning to get in touch with what you feel, want, and need
- Expressing yourself honestly based on how you are feeling, what you need, and what you'd like to happen
- Taking responsibility for how you feel rather than blaming someone else for making you feel a certain way
- Using "I" language rather than "you" language. Instead of saying, "You made me feel shitty when you decided to go on a date with her when I was sick," you say: "I felt hurt when you went on that date because I really wanted you to stay home and take care of me."

NVC is useful for people in open relationships for several reasons. It stresses a noncombative style of relating—one that is contrary to the way most people argue—to get people to practice empathy and kindness when they communicate with each other. The more relationships you have, the more processing of everyone's feelings you'll do; learning how to communicate without escalating into blame, judgment, and argument is essential. NVC pushes you to get to the heart of what you feel, and why, and to share it with the other person. It teaches you to own your emotions instead of making the other person at fault for them.

Honesty

Like consent, honesty is a key quality that distinguishes nonmonogamy from cheating. Unfortunately, dishonesty surrounds us. Government officials, business leaders, celebrities—many of them considered role models—are caught twisting the truth, misleading, covering up, stealing, and lying every day. So it is regrettable but perhaps understandable that the most prevalent and visible form of nonmonogamy in our society is both nonconsensual and dishonest. Cheating on one's spouse has become an integral part of our culture, and while it may not be openly supported, it is practiced by a staggering number of people.

Society teaches us that if we find ourselves attracted to or in love with someone other than our partner, or if we have sex or a relationship with them, we must keep it a secret. In fact, many people have a nearly unconscious compulsion to withhold even their nonmonogamous thoughts and desires from their partners, let alone disclose those actions. We need to let go of the notion that venturing beyond monogamy is wrong or shameful, or that it calls for us to behave dishonestly.

Honesty is crucial to creating and sustaining a positive and fulfilling open relationship. Without it, the relationship might survive for a while, but it will never thrive or be truly meaningful. When we tell the truth about who we are, what we need and want, and how we feel, it helps us feel connected to people and form deep bonds with them. Telling the truth is not always easy, especially when you feel that the disclosure will hurt someone you love. But withholding information to protect someone is not only unfair to them, it is counterproductive to the relationship.

> I really just say what is not being said. It is what you are not saying that is getting in the way of everything. —Dillon

Honesty is not just about engaging in ethical behavior and doing the right thing. It is a valuable tool for reassuring your partner and strengthening an open relationship. Many of the people I spoke to said that when their partners share information with them, they feel informed and in the loop. Knowing what's going on makes them feel more secure about their relationship and more connected to their partner. Many say that they feel the most insecure, jealous, and anxious when they don't know what is up. What often happens is that they use their imagination to fill in the blanks, fear and irrationality come into play, and they make something into what it is not or imagine the worst-case scenario.

Radical Honesty

Several people that I interviewed practice Radical Honesty or some of its tenets in their open relationships; it is also written about and taught within polyamory communities. Like Nonviolent Communication, Radical Honesty has spawned dozens of books, lectures, and workshops. The concept was developed by the psychologist Brad Blanton and first outlined in his book *Radical Honesty: How to Transform Your Life by Telling the Truth*. The premise is that most people develop roles that they present to the world which aren't truly who they are. As part of this role creation, people are not honest with their loved ones about who they are, things they've done, and what they think, feel, and want. This lack of honesty leads to unfulfilling, unsatisfying relationships, because the connections between people are based on phony behavior.

Blanton argues that to achieve true intimacy we must share everything, expose every lie and fiction, leave nothing unsaid, and not sugar-coat any of it. In one of his "levels" of truth telling, Blanton recommends that people "begin the practice of admitting how you feel when you feel it, speaking your secret judgments of others out loud, and constantly revealing your own petty and condescending ways."[4] Think of it as the opposite of biting your tongue, keeping it to yourself, or "not saying anything if you don't have anything nice to say." To practice Radical Honesty, you must speak everything regardless of how the person you're speaking to may react.

Some people who practice nonmonogamy believe strongly that Radical Honesty is a necessary component for a successful relationship. I appreciate some of Blanton's concepts. I believe we do create facades to please and impress others. I believe we must become more honest with ourselves and others to live authentically. However, I don't subscribe to Radical Honesty as a whole, and Blanton himself admits you have to do it completely or it doesn't work. I believe it is an egotistical and confrontational style of communication. It isn't fair or useful to share everything with someone who doesn't want to hear it, is not ready to hear it, or doesn't have the skills to process the information.

Tantra teachers Mark Michaels and Patricia Johnson, who coach couples about their relationships, have seen how Radical Honesty can be hurtful rather than helpful. Johnson says:

> It's often just brutal, and it encourages a nonrelational way of communicating that's totally self-involved. We've seen people use it as a club for beating up their partners. They'll say, "I'm just being honest," or "I'm just allowing you to know what my needs are or my hurts are." They're often completely oblivious about how that message is being received and have no willingness to take any responsibility for the damage they've done, because being "honest" gives them an excuse.[5]

When I asked them to name the most fundamental element of creating and sustaining a positive open relationship, Michaels said, "Honesty and the ability to communicate kindly." Nearly everyone lists honesty and communication as essentials; I asked him to elaborate on his conception of kind communication. He said this:

> Kindness is very hard. I'm certainly not always kind, but it's an ongoing process and an effort; I think that what it shows

is that the relationship matters and that your partner will try not to hurt you. Part of being in a relationship involves taking care of the other person. There can be excessive caretaking, and that can be very damaging, but I think that, in large part, the really unfortunate by-product of the human potential movement is that it's all about getting mine. It's not about us; it's all about me. I've seen enough of that to know how destructive it can be. If you're in a relationship with someone, you're in a sort of orbit. There has to be a kind of gravitational pull toward each other. If all of your focus is on yourselves, you're just going to fly off in different directions, and there's not going to be a relationship. I think a commitment to kindness can be the gravity that keeps you in orbit.[6]

Folks who practice Radical Honesty may see kindness as sugar-coating, but I believe it's a necessary component of compassionate communication.

Boundaries

Personal boundaries are what we use to define ourselves as separate from others, express our needs and wants, and set limits within relationships. When you have healthy boundaries, you recognize that you are an individual with your own wants, needs, and values. You don't take on other people's issues as your own or allow others to dictate your behavior based on what they want. You don't sacrifice your own desires and needs to please another person. You don't attempt to control someone else or allow yourself to be controlled. Boundaries are an important element in healthy relationships of all kinds, and open relationships are no exception.

Boundaries can be physical, sexual, or emotional/psychological. For example:

- Physical boundary: Don't touch me without my permission.
- Sexual boundary: Don't pinch my nipples during sex.
- Emotional boundary: Don't project your feelings onto me.

First you must determine what your boundaries are, and then you must be able to articulate them to your partner(s). Finally, you must be aware when someone does not respect your boundaries, and speak up for yourself. If you set a boundary and someone violates it, don't let it slide; that only sends the message *If you don't respect my boundaries, that's cool. I won't say anything. It's okay to disrespect my boundaries.*

For some people, emotional/psychological boundaries are the most complex and difficult to defend. Here's a hypothetical example. You go out with your friends and come home to your partner giddy and excited from a fun night. Your partner is angry. "I can't believe you went out and left me home alone! You're such a bitch! Then you come home and rub it in my face to make me feel worse!" *Without good personal boundaries*, you would apologize for going out and having a good time and for being bubbly when you walked through the door. You acknowledge that you're a bad girlfriend.

With good personal boundaries, you would recognize that your partner is feeling bad. You check yourself: Do I have the right to go out with my friends? Yes. Did I rub it in his face? No. You refuse to take on his feelings or to feel guilty about your night out. You recognize that something is pushing your partner's buttons, and that he's trying to make you feel bad instead of owning what's really going on. You tell him, "I can see that you're angry about me going out with friends tonight instead of being with you. I respect your feelings, but I did not do anything wrong. I was sharing my excitement with you, not deliberately trying to make you feel bad."

Learning to define good personal boundaries and respecting the boundaries of others are skills that may not have been modeled for you, or your partner, as you grew up. You may have to develop these skills.

Ultimately, boundaries are about clarity: being clear about who you are and what you need. If the line between you and your partner starts to blur, it's time to work on your boundaries.

Trust

Trust is a significant component in opening up a relationship to additional sexual and emotional partners. When a partner agrees to something you ask for and honors that agreement, it helps build your trust in them. Trust takes time to establish, but it leads to security. Many people in long-term relationships say that trust makes it easier to support and encourage their partners to explore

What the new model of open-ended marriage seeks to promote is risk-taking in trust; the warmth of loving without anxiety; the extension of affection; the excitement and pleasure of knowing sensuously a variety of other persons; the enrichment which personalities can contribute to each other; the joy of being fully alive in every encounter.
—RONALD MAZUR[7]

with other people. Trust becomes an antidote to jealousy, competitiveness, possessiveness, insecurity, and fear. The message is clear: when people trust their partners and trust in the strength of their relationships, they experience less anxiety in the presence of someone new. On the flip side, a lack of trust can lead to insecurity, doubt, and unhappiness.

Some people have difficulty trusting others because of unresolved issues from childhood or past relationships. No matter how trustworthy your behavior, someone who has a hard time trusting will still find it hard to trust you. If you know that trust is difficult for you, working on it can help you resolve some of the underlying issues and avert problems in your open relationships. Often a partner's paranoia, possessiveness, or jealousy can stem from a lack of trust. If your partner has trust issues, be patient, reassuring, and supportive; do not take on his insecurity by agreeing to unrealistic expectations or sharing his paranoia; encourage him to get help working on the issue.

Polyamory educator Anita Wagner believes that pacing yourself in a relationship can positively affect the trust level:

> Trust is based on knowing a person not just in what they say about themselves, but observing them as well. It takes a while to get to know someone really well. The newer your relationship, the less substantial the foundation for it, in terms of really knowing and trusting each other. Now, there's a case to be made for the opposite: you can learn to trust that person, see them go out [with someone else], come back, continue to do right by your relationship, continue to be invested in it. So trust can be built that way too, but there has to be a good balance. Pacing yourself early in relationships helps to keep things stable and helps prevent the big blowups, the big crash-and-burns.[8]

Wagner makes an important point: don't rush the process of building trust. The more deeply you trust someone, the easier it will be to take the leap of faith with her as you explore possibilities beyond monogamy.

Fidelity and Commitment

One of the values most strongly associated with monogamy and traditional marriage is fidelity. Every day, in their wedding vows, spouses promise to be faithful to each other and to forsake all others. Most folks assume that if you're in a nonmonogamous relationship, you're being unfaithful by definition. Nonmonogamous people have tossed out the "forsaking all others" part, but that doesn't mean they reject the notion of fidelity.

Although monogamy and fidelity have become intertwined in cultural definitions, fidelity ultimately means believing strongly in your love and in your relationship, and *keeping your promises*. If the statistics on cheating are accurate, keeping your promises is something monogamous people have a tough time doing. Nonmonogamous relationships are built not on vows of exclusivity but on the agreements people make and honor; therefore, fidelity is an essential part of nonmonogamy.

There is a false assumption that open relationships are less committed than monogamous ones. This is because nonmonogamous people often make commitments in the absence of the legal documents, state recognition, and financial rewards and benefits that come with a marital commitment. They often do not have the acknowledgment, support, or acceptance of friends and families. In the absence of such external validation, they are bound together by their faith in each other and by their daily words and deeds.

Of course, self-awareness, communication, healthy boundaries, trust, fidelity, and commitment aren't the only values that make open relationships work. People in open relationships also embrace respect, generosity, freedom, and authenticity. One last quality that cannot go unmentioned in any discussion of open relationships is *compersion*, a concept that may be new to many readers. Compersion is taking joy in your partner's pleasure or happiness with another partner. For some, compersion has an erotic component: they get turned on watching, imagining, or hearing about their partner's sexual experiences. Some practitioners of polyamory think of compersion as the opposite of jealousy, or at least the antidote to jealousy. Given the problems (and drama) ignited by jealousy, you can see how compersion can go a long way toward creating a foundation for pleasure and generosity in any relationship. Read more about compersion in Chapter 13.

Chapter 5

Partnered Nonmonogamy

THIS SECTION OF THE BOOK is devoted to different styles of open relationships. While I name and define these styles, they are not meant to be rigid categories, but rather a loose framework from which you can start to build your unique relationships.

Partnered nonmonogamy is a style for committed couples who want a relationship that is erotically nonmonogamous, where each partner can be involved with other people for sex, BDSM, or other erotic activities. The BDSM play may or may not include genital sex. I make this distinction because some BDSM does not involve sex. For some who enjoy BDSM, many activities—for example, flogging, piercing, and hot wax—are intense, erotic, satisfying, and even orgasmic without any sexual contact. Whether or not BDSM play with other partners includes genital sex is something that every couple needs to negotiate. Your definition of sex, or of BDSM, may not encompass some of the activities you engage in with others—for example, crossdressing, foot worship, or a particular fetish.

Experiences with other people may occur once or be recurring, but they are generally considered temporary, casual, commitment-free, and nonromantic. The primary focus of your time and energy is your committed relationship, not entering a serious relationship with anyone else. If you have fantasized together about bringing a third person into your bed for a night, if you want to have a casual fling (or two) while you're out of town, or if you'd like a sex or BDSM playmate whom you see regularly, then this style may be your ideal form of nonmonogamy.

You and your partner might choose partnered nonmonogamy if:

- you want to have sex/BDSM with others but your relationship remains the priority
- you have no interest in additional partners for anything but sex or BDSM and possibly friendship
- you want to fulfill a fantasy that involves group sex, multiple-partner sex, or a group BDSM scene
- you want to have sex or play with a person of a different gender than your primary partner
- you want to express a part of yourself sexually with someone other than your primary partner, perhaps to fulfill certain sexual or kinky desires, needs, or fantasies
- you want to explore a sexual, BDSM, or other activity that your partner has no interest, experience, or skill in
- you want to explore a specific role or power dynamic (Top/bottom, Dominant/submissive) with someone other than your primary partner

I know two men in a relationship who are committed to one another to be sexually exclusive, with one exception: each is allowed to hook up with other men at bathhouses or at the gym, provided it goes no further than mutual masturbation. This couple doesn't consider masturbation "sex," so they think of themselves as "monogamous with benefits."

David and Sadie also consider themselves monogamous, although they do BDSM play and some sexual activity with others. "We can play with other people, but no sex. By no sex, I mean no vaginal or anal intercourse. There can be genital contact, orgasms, fisting, penetration with toys," Sadie says. David says, "Playing with different people provides different experiences. Playing with your spouse can bring in different, more complicated emotions. Playing with close friends and others allows for different types of emotions and connections, but not necessarily baggage that you have to take home."

Jason makes a clear distinction between his relationship and his other activities: "I definitely have a single significant other. While I certainly fuck/play with other people, there's a distinct boundary of 'home' and 'extracurricular.' My girlfriend is the person I live with, work with, spend most of my time with, and most importantly, love."

Shari and Eli have been married for seven years, and their marriage has been nonmonogamous from the start. Shari says:

I love the freedom of being able to be this sexual and not having to lie about this aspect of myself in order to have a mate who loves me for who and what I am. It's brilliant that he loves me for this aspect of my sexuality, instead of in spite of it. We each needed a partner who really, truly, wasn't possessive or jealous. I love the incredible bonding that occurs with good sex, and being able to spread joy and fun and pleasure. I love knowing my husband is having fun with others; our sex is always better when we are alone again. The more men I fuck, the more I love my husband.

When they first got together, Shari had a long-term male lover whom Eli wasn't comfortable with: "She still had strong feelings for him that I found somewhat threatening, as they seemed to transcend mere sexual desire." He asked her to stop seeing him, and she agreed, but the issue remained on the table:

For the first five years, Eli asked me to not see my lover, to whom I was still very attached. I didn't think I should have to do it, since my relationship with my lover preceded my marriage. However,

I wanted to prove to him as well as myself that I was trustworthy and committed to my relationship with my husband. We had a serious discussion about it at least twice a year for those five years, as we figured out just where our needs lay and built intimacy and trust. Five years later, I still wanted to see my lover, but I had worked through all of my issues surrounding my not seeing him, so the charge was off. My husband and I were able to have a conversation about our needs and where they differed and what we were going to do to address them, calmly, without recriminations or guilt tripping. As life would have it, my husband had come to the understanding that he, too, needed a partner who could go places with him that I just couldn't go, in order that some of his core needs could be met.

Eli says, "Ultimately, I came to realize that she needed a more 'vanilla' kind of sexual and emotional involvement than I could provide. I am now at peace with the satisfaction she derives from her encounters with him." While both Shari and Eli are kinky, they have desires which don't overlap. Eli is her Dominant, but realized he wanted to play with submissives who were more experienced. Shari likes to switch roles and is also bisexual, plus she yearns for a dynamic that isn't power-driven, which Eli can't give her. Their nonmonogamy helps them get their needs met by each other and other people.

Partnered nonmonogamy may also be a good compromise for a heterosexual male crossdresser and his wife. Let's say D likes to dress occasionally in women's clothes, and crossdressing sexually arouses him. He has fantasies of someone helping to dress him, which may or may not also involve sexual contact. His wife supports his desire but has no interest in participating in his dressing fantasy. So, they talk about it and agree that he can attend a crossdressing event, and, if he meets another woman, they can have a dressing session. The one rule: no sexual play at all. This is fine with him, since he finds the experience incredibly intimate and intense and prefers to masturbate on his own afterward.

Ovate, a crossdresser in his thirties who's enlisted in the military, says, "My wife is okay with my crossdressing. She did research on her own to try to understand it better. She's a very cerebral person. But it was never something that she could enjoy with me, and she could never be comfortable enough with it to be sexual in any way. And while I know this isn't true for all crossdressers, it is a very sexual thing for me." One of the benefits he gets from his open relationship is a chance to have friends and other partners with whom he can crossdress.

For this style to be successful for you, you should be pretty good at having a no-strings-attached sexual, BDSM, or other erotic experience. You must be very clear about your boundaries. If you have trouble distinguishing lust from love, or if you easily get attached to or fall in love with someone after a sexual experience, then keeping sex "on the side" may be too challenging for you. Some people can't just fuck a person and walk away. They need to get to know them first and make a connection to even consider getting naked with them. For these folks, attraction and chemistry aren't enough; the courtship of compliments, seduction, and dating all contribute to their desire, and this focused attention is necessary for a sexual relationship to work. If this rings true for you, you may want to consider creating room for dating, as long as it remains either casual or secondary, in your ideal style.

Potential Issues and Conflicts in This Style

In addition to the feelings and conflicts covered above and in later chapters—jealousy, possessiveness, resentment, insecurity, shame and guilt, time management problems, and when rules are broken—here are some potential conflicts that may arise that are specific to partnered nonmonogamy:

Sex or Play Becomes More

The most important aspect of this style is the commitment by both partners to make the primary relationship central and give all outside
experiences lower priority. To achieve this, you must keep your physical,
emotional, and psychological investment in other people low. You can
take steps to prevent yourself from becoming too attached to an outside
partner, such as limiting your communication and social contact with
them; expending only a small amount of time on outside activities; and
spending a limited amount of money and resources on outside activities.
However, sex becomes something more sometimes, and people develop
deeper feelings. And sometimes people fall in love. Once you open up
your relationship, this is always a risk, since the way people connect and
the depth of emotions that arise cannot be predicted.

If deeper feelings emerge, the person having these feelings
must first of all be honest with their partner about them. This is not
a time to engage in denial or to protect your partner from being
hurt. You owe it to your partner to be up front about what's going
on. This can feel like a serious betrayal to him or her, and that must
be acknowledged.

The outcome of this conflict depends completely on the two of
you. Some couples break up over this issue, because it is a breach of
their intent to remain emotionally monogamous. Others agree to stay
together as long as the relationship with the new person is ended.
Others renegotiate their relationship to accommodate this change and
explore a different form of nonmonogamy: polyamory, which allows for
multiple loving relationships. (See Chapter 7 for more on polyamory.)

An "On the Side" Desire Becomes Central

If the phrase "you want to explore a sexual, BDSM, or other activity
that your primary partner has no interest, experience, or skill in"
describes you, beware a particular pitfall. When you discover a desire
that doesn't fit in your relationship, ask yourself how critical this activ-

ity is to your identity and overall sexual satisfaction. Is it something that your partner must be into for you to be truly intimate, or are you okay sharing this with someone else? Maybe all you need is your primary partner's acknowledgment of this facet of your erotic life, and her support and her blessing to explore it. Similarly, you must determine if engaging in this activity only occasionally will be fulfilling for you, since within the partnered nonmonogamy model most of your time and energy is spent on your primary relationship.

Sometimes only when you start to explore the desire do you realize that what you thought you could do just "on the side" is actually much more important to you than that. You may find out that doing it occasionally is not enough, or it has moved up on the list of important things in your life, or it is something you want to be able to do with your partner. For instance, a married man might realize his attraction to men and come out as bisexual. He believes he's content to remain married to his wife and have sex with men on the side. However, as he begins to explore sexual relationships with men, he realizes that he really wants his life partner to be a man. In a scenario such as this, you may want to explore polyamory instead (see Chapter 7), or else end the relationship.

The Primary Relationship Gets Neglected

It's very easy to be distracted by all the good feelings that come with having sex with someone for the first time, or getting to know a new sexual partner. You can get caught up in the giddy feelings, become focused on the outside sex and the outside partners, and take your primary relationship for granted. Don't forget that no matter how long you've been together, your primary partner needs attention, nurturing, and love. Problems in the primary relationship will not go away just by avoiding them or keeping busy with extracurricular sex.

Some people say that for partnered nonmonogamy to be successful, you must separate your emotions from sex or keep sex and love absolutely separate. I respectfully disagree. You can be emotionally present and connected to a person other than your primary partner and you can have feelings for her or him. You can have deep, intense, soul-shattering sex together. The point is that your intention is to have sex or do BDSM, to enjoy each other's bodies, but not to pursue a relationship beyond that. If you are clear about your intentions up front and you honor your primary relationship, the experiences you have outside it can genuinely enhance it.

PROFILE: BEN AND CLAIRE

"We're sexual adventurists."

BEN, 48, AND CLAIRE, 43, have been together for eight and a half years and married for nearly seven. Claire grew up in a small town in the Midwest and began practicing nonmonogamy in college: "I had up to five boyfriends at a time. It seemed natural. Unless someone requested exclusivity, I assumed that the relationship was open. With some, I spoke openly about seeing others. With others, I never mentioned it. Some were married. Some had other girlfriends. I had deep feelings for every one." Ben's first foray into nonmonogamy was also in college, though he considers it unsuccessful. "I had a girlfriend in college who had multiple other boyfriends and it was fine for her to see them and be with them. Then I started seeing someone else and [my existing girlfriend] couldn't deal with it. She said, 'I don't think we should see each other anymore because of this. I got really upset when you were with this other woman.' So I broke up with the other person, but my girlfriend kept seeing other people. I spent a lot of time accepting her double standard, and that was very unhappy-making for me." Later in life, Ben was in a monogamous relationship for 12 years, including seven years of marriage, but never found it satisfying. He didn't cheat, but he did go to strip clubs to get lap dances and felt very guilty about it. He says he felt guilty about his sexuality in general.

Ben and Claire got engaged the morning after going to a swing club together. "At that time, we were doing only the most casual exploration of interacting with others—light touch and nothing more," Ben says. "Still, it was clear that we both viewed sexuality as something to be explored, and the direct experience of exploring sex together kind of sealed the deal for us. Sexuality and sexual exploration has been one of the central parts of our relationship all along. So, the whole discussion about monogamy and nonmonogamy is something that we've talked about from day one in one form or another." Today, they consider themselves pair-bonded and nonmonogamous; they have sex with other people and may have friendships, but their only partnered relationship is with each other. Ben notes: "I'm not really that interested in polyamory in the sense of wanting to have other really deep emotional relationships with people. I definitely want to be friends with the people that we play with, and there's definitely an element of love that comes in some of the relationships that we have. But for me, she's my partner and my focus and it's just too much of an emotional dissipation for me to think about getting really involved with other people."

They socialize in many different alternative communities among swingers, kinky people, and sex-positive folks. When they have sex with other people, they almost always do it together: "By and large, we really enjoy group energy and being together in these settings. The few times I've gone off on my own, I've missed having her there. We always talk about these experiences, and the ability to be open about them is very important," Ben says.

As for the rules they have agreed to, Claire says: "Always check in. Anyone can veto at any moment. No abandonment allowed, no 'I have a date tonight, so you take care of yourself.'" For this couple, sexual adventures play a significant role in their relationship: "The most appealing thing is that we facilitate each other's individual sexual evolution.

Thus, our sexual life together is forever evolving. Our beef with traditional monogamy is that it puts a cap on that part of a person's evolution.
We find that sexual adventuring has a profound effect on deepening
our bond. We have learned so much about ourselves and each other
and have developed incredible trust through our sexual experiences."

Chapter 6

Swinging

THE UNIQUE HISTORY, traditions, culture, etiquette, philosophies, and communities of swingers are beyond the scope of this book and have been documented in many publications. Swingers can practice any number of open relationship styles, though the majority of them likely identify most with the style outlined in the previous chapter, partnered nonmonogamy. Indeed, much of what I discussed in that chapter can be applied to swinging. However, swinging warrants its own chapter because swingers have their own distinct identities and subcultures. When a person identifies as a swinger, it's not just about being nonmonogamous. Swinging is about the context in which they practice their nonmonogamy, the way they socialize, and their community. It's about, as many refer to it, the *lifestyle*.

Not all swingers are the same, and each swinger community has a unique culture; however, the majority of swingers share similar beliefs and attitudes, and certain social norms and etiquette can be seen across different swinger communities.

Sex with other couples causes us to be more intimate with each other. It helps me communicate openly with my partner and dig

deep into my feelings, which is something hard for me to do. After
going to a swinger party and having sex with others, the sex we
have with each other is intimate and amazing. —Janie

Beliefs and Attitudes

Swingers come from all walks of life and all areas of the country, but
the majority are white, middle or upper-middle class, married, middle-
aged professionals. Most of the men identify as heterosexual and the
women as heterosexual, bi-curious, or bisexual. Very few gay, lesbian,
queer, or transgendered people identify as swingers. Swingers emphasize the social, fun aspect of what they do and are generally discreet
about their lifestyle. Although their behavior falls outside traditional
monogamy, they are not a politicized community and rarely see themselves as radical or nontraditional.

The majority of swingers consider themselves emotionally monogamous and sexually nonmonogamous. They view sex outside their
primary relationship very differently from sex with their spouse; they
see it as casual—"sport sex" or "recreational sex." In her book *Recreational
Sex*, Patti Thomas, editor of several popular swingers' magazines, writes:

> To swingers, *physical acts of sexual pleasure* with someone you
> respect, just for pleasure, and *making love* to one's lifetime
> partner, are two distinctly different things.[1]

As David says, "Sex can be casual, but tends to be with those we
know and have some connection with, though not in a committed
way."

Swingers adhere to very specific rules and etiquette—both spoken
and unspoken. Clubs and events are geared toward the couple as a
unit, and the emphasis is always on couples. In fact, at many swingers'
events, when you register and receive a name tag, the tag lists both

your name and your spouse's. Usually, the only singles allowed at swingers' spaces are women; rarely are single men welcome. There is a particularly problematic double standard at work in most swingers' spaces: while women are encouraged to be sexual with other women, male/male eroticism, desire, and sex is taboo. When swingers talk about sex, they usually mean intercourse, and many swingers are sexually conservative. For example, I have been to parties where there is little or no anal sex, BDSM, use of sex toys, or much of anything besides vaginal intercourse.

Swinging Styles

Within swinging, there are different options and practices, depending on what you're comfortable with and what you want. Like other open relationship styles, there is room for people to play at their own speed and do what feels right for them.

Soft Swinging

In soft swinging, two couples have sex in the same room, each person with their own spouse or partner, with no intention of switching partners for intercourse. Instead, they watch each other; the women may kiss, touch, fondle, or have oral sex with each other, or each woman may do these things with the man who is not her partner. Some couples start out doing soft swinging as a way to test the water and have the experience without going "all the way." For others, soft swinging isn't a stepping stone, it is the way they swing: they want to be sexual in some way with other people but have agreed not to have intercourse with anyone else.

Swinging with One

Because single women are allowed at most clubs and events, but not single men, couples often play together with another woman. Sometimes, if the single woman is a lesbian or bisexual, she hooks up with a couple but is sexual only with the woman. A couple may also split up for the evening so each partner can play separately, but only after making sure they have their partner's consent. This gives a man the opportunity to play with a couple without his female partner, but usually he only has sex with the woman in the couple.

Swinging with Another Couple

Many couples primarily have sex with other couples, although usually, again, the men are not sexual together. Swinging with another couple, rather than a single person, assures some couples that there's less chance for potential romance or unwanted drama. We're married, they're married, we're on the same page: no strings attached, our commitment is to our families. One of the tricky things about playing with another couple is that each partner must be attracted to or interested in having sex with the opposite partner. If you and your spouse have very different taste in sexual partners, a match may not be easy to find. Say you have agreed not to split up for sex play and your partner suggests a couple you don't like. You have to turn them down, which may disappoint your partner. Most swingers agree that all participants need to be into the scenario for it to work; no one should "take one for the team" so their partner can have a good time. Swinger couples may socialize with other swinger couples outside of events, but usually not in a romantic way.

Group Swinging

Swinging in a group is exactly like it sounds: having sex with multiple partners or couples at once; this is more like group sex or an orgy. When some people think of swingers, images of wild orgies may come to mind, but in reality only a small percentage of swingers regularly have group sex; there is a much greater emphasis on couple-to-couple contact.

Social Swinging

Some swingers are attracted to the community and clubs for the fun, free, open social atmosphere and less for the sex. They may have sex with other people occasionally or rarely. More often, they love to flirt, touch, watch others, get turned on, then retire to their own room and have sex with each other. Terry Gould, who studied swinger communities in the mid-nineties for his book *The Lifestyle*, met a couple in British Columbia who had been in the swinging scene for about five years. Gould writes: "Most of the time, they said, they didn't even swing. They just enjoyed being in a close-knit crowd of married people where the boundary between friendship and sex was a titillating line to be openly approached, not a wall to sneak around in deceit."[2]

Community

Swinging is steeped in community, and most swingers belong to a local group, attend social clubs, parties, and events, and choose their additional partners from within swinger communities. In fact, some swing only at swinger-specific clubs and events. Because swinging is very couples-focused and includes only single women, if you're a single guy you're likely to have a tough time finding swingers' spaces that welcome you. (I have known two single friends to hook up and present themselves as a couple to attend functions together.) If you live near a large city (and even some not-so-large cities), chances are there is a swingers' club or organization near you. A quick search on the Internet can provide you with enough information to get started. (Also see the Resource Guide at the end of this book.) An entire industry of clubs, events, vacations, personals, and websites exists for swingers. For some groups, you must attend an orientation or meet the leaders before you're invited to a party. Other groups and small swingers' parties at private homes may be more underground and require that you know a member to get in.

For some swingers, swinging is central to their social life—it is their primary identity and community. Others may float in and out of the scene or only occasionally attend parties. Many swingers develop long-term relationships with other couples, socializing and traveling together away from swingers' events.

Etiquette

As with all sexual experiences, you need to approach swinging with a clear sense of your limits—what's okay and what's not. Because swingers are a close-knit group, people who don't respect others' boundaries or don't follow the rules get weeded out pretty quickly. The majority of swingers are dedicated to being polite, respectful, and well-behaved; consent is very important, and if they sense that one spouse is being dragged along, that couple is not going to get a lot of dates.

Once you decide what style of swinging you'd like to try, you should decide where you want to do it. Swingers' parties are commonly referred to as "on premises" or "off premises." An "on premises" event means that there are spaces where you can have sex on-site at the house, club, hotel, or other venue. So if you meet someone you like, you don't have to leave to hook up. These spaces may be public (a large ballroom at a hotel), semipublic (multiple rooms without doors, or cubbies with curtains), private (rooms with doors that shut), or some combination. An "off premises" event is a party where you can meet other swingers but you must go elsewhere if you want to have sex. An off premises party may be held at a local bar or club, for example, where the atmosphere is sexually charged; flirting and petting are fine, but if you want to go beyond that you have to go to someone's place. Some events take place at hotels, where you can socialize in large public spaces and retire to your room for sexual action.

Potential Issues and Conflicts in This Style

The conflicts that come up with partnered nonmonogamy apply also to swinging, especially if sex becomes more than casual and recreational or you neglect your primary relationship in favor of swinging. Because the swingers' world is so couples-centric, there is a built-in expectation that your primary relationship should be the focus. Couples come to swinging with the intention to maintain their relationship while having sex for fun and pleasure, but that doesn't mean that things cannot go awry. If you can find swingers who have similar intentions and goals, you're ahead of the game.

A potential issue may come up with bi-curious or bisexual men. It used to be that male bisexuality was forbidden in nearly every swingers' space, but things have changed a great deal. Today, there are swinger communities that support male/male attraction and sex, and some events even cater to bisexual women *and* bisexual men. If you are a bi-curious or bisexual man and you are concerned about whether you will be accepted, I recommend you do some research to find bi-friendly swingers near you. Similarly, if you are outside the core demographic of swingers, know that there are swingers' groups for people of color, urban swingers' parties, and events that cater to kinky swingers or swingers under 40. If it's swinging you want, you can probably find a community within this large subculture that suits you.

PROFILE: AGNES AND RAYMOND

"We trust ourselves, therefore we trust each other."

AGNES IS A 55-YEAR-OLD sales representative with one of the largest cosmetic companies in the US. Raymond is 55 and works for a public utility company. They live in Iowa and have been married for 20 years.

This is the second marriage for both of them; during their courtship and the beginning of their marriage, they were monogamous.

About six years ago, after 14 years of marriage, they were sharing erotic fantasies with each other and Raymond asked Agnes if she had ever had a fantasy about being with another woman; Agnes said yes. They agreed they wanted to try to fulfill the fantasy, but they had no idea how to do it. Agnes says, "We made a trip to Kansas City and answered an ad placed by a woman in a weekly alternative newspaper. She came to our hotel room and the three of us had sex. Okay, so we had to pay her, but it was still fun!" After that positive experience, they found a swingers' club closer to home, then went to a "swingers' week" at a resort. For Agnes, the transition from monogamy to swinging was a long process:

"When we first went on vacation to an adult resort—Hedonism II in Jamaica—it wasn't difficult to go to the beach and get naked, because we were already nudists. What was difficult was grasping the concept that we were there to have sex with other people. I felt immense pressure being put on me to 'find someone to have sex with.' Raymond thought he was giving me the freedom to find women or couples I was comfortable around. I thought that everyone I talked to, had coffee with, or met for dinner, it automatically meant we were going to hook up. Way too much pressure. We eventually found a couple that helped us get over our newbie jitters. Once we relaxed, we met lots of new friends and had a great time; some new friends we had sex with, some we didn't. It was definitely a new situation for both of us and we learned a lot from that first vacation.

"After that vacation, followed by more swinger events, we talked at length about how we felt, what we liked and disliked about the event and the couples we met. The idea of sharing each other with another person, and then talking about it, was scary at first. Seeing your partner with someone else having a good time brings up those green-eyed jealousy monsters. We talked a lot about the strength of our commitment to each other and how much each other's happiness meant to both of us. We talked about how we are married, have a good marriage, and plan to stay that way. We trusted ourselves, therefore we trusted each other. We've grown to like the idea that we both have the freedom to pursue sexual pleasure from other people, within the boundaries we've set. Since we've had these outside-of-marriage experiences with other people, we discuss topics more openly with each other. Nothing is off limits: feelings, ideas for sex, money, retirement, travel, health—you name it, we talk about it. By trusting ourselves and each other, stepping out of the 'monogamy box' has been very liberating for us."

Chapter 7

Polyamory

TO DISTINGUISH POLYAMORY from swinging and partnered non-monogamy, poly relationships are usually characterized as "sexual and loving," a shorthand way of saying that polyamory involves not just sex, but *emotional* relationships. But based on my research, "sexual and loving" doesn't capture the nuances and complexities of polyamorous relationships, or the way in which polyamory not only rejects mainstream models but expands our ideas about what constitutes a relationship. I would define polyamory as the desire for or the practice of maintaining multiple significant, intimate relationships simultaneously. These relationships may encompass many elements, including love, friendship, closeness, emotional intimacy, recurring contact, commitment, affection, flirting, romance, desire, erotic contact, sex, and a spiritual connection.

Now, some swingers and partnered nonmonogamists might argue that while their outside relationships are primarily sex- or BDSM-based, there is also an emotional connection or some other element from the list above. Setting up false dichotomies such as sexual versus emotional, casual versus committed, or playful versus serious just gets us into a whole heap of trouble. Some people I interviewed conceptualized and constructed their relationships in all the ways I've just discussed but say they aren't polyamorous. Two people may define their relationships in very similar ways, yet one calls herself nonmonogamous and the other polyamorous. Remember: don't get stuck on the labels if they feel confining to you; define your relationships on your terms.

Some polyamorous people have strong ties to a local poly organization or community, a broader poly community, or both. Others may not identify with any community, for a variety of reasons: there is no organized group in their area, they have no interest in a broader community, or they don't feel they are part of one.

Beliefs and Attitudes

There is no single way to be polyamorous. Some poly people pass judgment on others, saying, "Well, she's not *really* poly," but that kind of attitude is counterproductive. The beauty of polyamory is that it frees you from arbitrary lines and limits, so why construct new ones? Indulge in the freedom to define polyamory and your relationships however you want. Now, that said, there are some similarities among polyamorous people in their basic beliefs and practices. Not every polyamorous individual shares all the values discussed below, but they were echoed again and again by the people I interviewed.

Many polyamorous people believe that it's unrealistic to expect that one person can fulfill all your needs. Therapist and author Daphne Rose Kingma cleverly describes our unreasonable fairy-tale expectations about relationships:

> When we fall in love, we're not just saying, "My, what a wonderful mind you have, it'll be a joy to talk with you over the next fifty years." What we're actually saying is "My, what a wonderful mind you have; I'm also expecting you to be a great lover, a great father, a wonderful Friday night date, my

comforter in times of sorrow, my social sidekick, my political compatriot, the person my parents will dote on, as well as my guru, my emotional crying towel, and my First Personal National Bank."[1]

One of the reasons relationships fail is because we do have unrealistic expectations going into them, fueled by myths about "the one" true love who's going to be our "everything." Polyamorous people recognize this fallacy and respect each person's capabilities and limits when it comes to what they can give. Instead of attempting to change someone, demanding that they be something they're not, or resenting them for not being Superpartner, poly people have multiple relationships so as to fulfill more of their sexual and emotional needs.

Let's say you're involved with someone and you develop feelings for another person. People who practice monogamy believe they must make a decision: squash the feelings and desires this new person has stirred in you and remain faithful to your current sweetheart, or break up to pursue a relationship with the new person. People who practice polyamory don't feel compelled to make it an either/or situation. That doesn't mean that everyone who comes along is fair game, but the possibility is open without having to end one relationship to pursue another.

As a group, polyamorous people have the courage to think outside the box of monogamy and to live outside the box. They recognize the importance of growth, for themselves as individuals, for their partners, and for their relationships. In general, they actively engage with their partners and work on their relationships; after all, it's pretty difficult to coast or to be on automatic pilot with more than one person. Many of the polyamorous people I interviewed said that one should allow a relationship to become whatever it will become. In other words, don't attempt to define it or limit it; instead, let the relationship evolve organically wherever it's going to go. For example:

*In a monogamous world, if you have somebody that you love to
kiss and you're not dating anyone else, there's pressure to figure
out if you're going to take it to the next level or if you're not going
to go there anymore. I have friends that I really enjoy kissing, and
that's it. I get to let those relationships be exactly what they are,
and that feels really comfortable to me.* —Ruby Grace

You might try polyamory if:

- you want to have multiple relationships and define those relationships on your terms
- you have the desire and capacity to love, share emotional and sexual intimacy, and commit to more than one partner
- you don't want to limit yourself to "just sex" from your additional relationships
- you want to explore different sexual or relationship dynamics with people of different genders
- you want certain erotic and emotional desires, needs, and fantasies fulfilled by different partners

Styles and Elements of Polyamory

Hierarchical Poly, or "One Primary Plus"

The ways in which people practice polyamory are unique and entirely specific to them. There is no formula for polyamory. But poly people generally adhere to one of two models: hierarchical and nonhierarchical. Consider which style feels more appropriate for you or fits with your goals.

Some poly people structure their relationships hierarchically, and they consider one relationship primary. A primary partner can be considered primary for a variety of reasons: the relationship is more central or significant than others; you live together; you make major life decisions together; you share resources and finances; you jointly own property or a business; you raise children together; you have made a formal commitment, such as marriage, domestic partnership, or handfasting; you are fluid-bonded (you share bodily fluids with each other without barriers); or you have been together longer than your other relationships.

Each partner in the primary couple can have one or more partners, but the additional partners are considered secondary, tertiary, or nonprimary. These nonprimary partners may be single or partnered with others, short-term or ongoing, sexual or romantic, or some combination; the constant is that they are considered secondary to the primary relationship. This style can work for you if you are currently in a relationship you consider to be primary and desire other partners, but no more primaries.

The benefit of designating one partner primary is that it's clear which relationship has priority over the others. Hierarchy can help define and bring structure to nontraditional relationships for which we have few models, providing an outline of your expectations in terms of the time and energy you're willing to give to the relationship. For some people, having a primary partner is like having a "home base," one person who is there for the long haul and with whom you have a shared history. The One Primary Plus style of polyamory honors what some scientists consider our natural instinct to pair-bond, while allowing room for other relationships as well.

Primary or nonprimary status does not have to be reciprocal. John may be Sue's primary partner, but Sue may be John's secondary partner. However, it is important to be clear in communicating your expectations so that a relationship doesn't feel unbalanced to one of the partners.

Some of the people I spoke to resisted the idea of hierarchy, but acknowledged that in many ways one of their partners was primary. They believe that their primary relationships don't fit what they see as the standard definitions of "primary." Claire said that she and her partner Dillon are primary in some ways, but not in the typical ones:

Naming Our Partners

Here are all the different names the people I interviewed gave to the significant others in their lives:

spouse

spice (plural of spouse)

custodial spouse

spouseling

wife

husband

legal husband

spiritual husband

co-husband

co-wife

nonhusband #1

partner

primary partner

life partner

live-in partner

platonic life partner

former partner

nonprimary partner

secondary partner

tertiary partner

partner in crime

significant other

other significant other (OSO)

lover

primary lover

sweetie

girlfriend

ex-girlfriend

boyfriend

former girlfriend/ boyfriend

boygirlfriend

steady beau

main squeeze

part-time lover

fuck buddy

make-out buddy

casual partner

friend

best friend

very good friend

horizontal friend

swinger friend

friend with benefits

Daddy

Uncle

Sir

Master

slave

slave brother

sister

boy

girl

boi

play partner

Dominant

submissive

pet

soul mate

secret agent lover man

sex toy

LDR (long distance relationship)

"I think when most people declare someone as their primary, they are declaring that they are no longer operating as a free agent in their romantic life, dating life and social life... In a lot of ways, Dillon and I function very independently."

Multiple Primaries or Multipartner Groups

Some people have more than one primary partner. Together these people form a unit—most often a triad or a quad—whose members are committed to each other. Because the configurations for these multipartner relationships are quite varied and they are considered types of polyfidelity, I devote an entire chapter to them (Chapter 9, Polyfidelity).

Nonprimary Partners

Sarah Sloane, a BDSM educator from the Washington, DC, area, teaches workshops on polyamory around the country. In her class Polyamory for Nonprimary Partners, she points out that one of the positive aspects of nonprimary relationships is that you can "add someone's presence to your life when it might not otherwise be possible—like, if you'd kill each other if you spent more than three consecutive days together."[2] Hers is a great point, and it's a good example of how polyamory questions the way relationships are supposed to be. Creating a secondary relationship flies in the face of the myth that if you love someone, you will want to spend all your time with him, live with him, be with him forever. Well, that's not always the case.

Although she doesn't use the terms *primary*, *nonprimary*, or *polyamory*, Daphne Rose Kingma, in *The Future of Love*, notes the widespread assumption that all relationships should model traditional marriage—they must be daily, domestic, exclusive, and forever.[3] She makes the case throughout her book that not all relationships are what she calls "marriage clones," but this raises an important point: while polyamory is a new relationship model, the primary relationship still has certain expectations and models to draw from, whereas nonprimary relationships have no existing blueprints. There are no agreed-upon rules or guidelines for how much time, energy, money, sex, or emotional support to give your secondary girlfriend, long-distance lover, or once-a-month friend with benefits. The familiar example of having a mistress or an affair is not comparable, because that is an entirely different dynamic based not on consent and negotiation but on lying and secrecy. Nonprimary relationships are an area within polyamory where you must break a lot of new ground to find a balance. As a result, some of the trickiest relationships to negotiate and nurture are nonprimary ones.

As with all the relationship styles, there are benefits and challenges to nonprimary relationships. Sloane sums up some of them: "Being a secondary partner can be special, like you're the exciting date night in an otherwise mundane week. But because you may not share in each other's lives on a daily basis, there can also be a sense of 'unreality' or a lack of intimacy." It's true that as a secondary, you may feel less connected to all facets of your partner's life. On the plus side, however, Sloane believes that being involved with someone who has a primary partner gives her the opportunity to observe her partner in a different relationship dynamic and learn a great deal from it. Whatever the dynamic, we must start by legitimizing, valuing, and respecting all of our relationships, whether primary, nonprimary, or something else entirely.

Nonhierarchical Polyamory

In nonhierarchical polyamory, no single relationship is considered primary. Each relationship is different and unique. They may all be equally important or they may vary greatly in terms of time, energy, commitment, and significance, but they are not ordered by priority. For poly people who intentionally choose not to create a hierarchy, a nonhierarchical approach is usually part of their overall personal philosophy.

Lynn acknowledges the practicality of hierarchy, but ultimately rejects it: "When you start talking about someone as your primary and actually believe in those categories, I think that limits the ways a relationship can evolve. I've got this thing about labels. I try not to use them if I can help it."

This style can work for you if you simply don't believe in hierarchy or feel that hierarchy is oppressive; if you don't consider one of your relationships to be any more primary or significant than any other; or if you believe each relationship is different and should be treated as such. Some people may prefer not to use hierarchical language, but may still designate one relationship as more important than the others.

I feel differently about all of my lovers. They each touch a different part of me. They nurture different aspects of myself. Even different sexual aspects of myself. Some are more emotional, some more intellectual, some more physical, some quite spiritual. —Beth

Solo Polyamory

For some poly folk hierarchy is not an issue, because they neither have nor want to have a primary partner. These folks, whom I call solo polyamorists, face their own set of issues, which I discuss in Chapter 8, Solo Polyamory.

Nonsexual Poly Relationships

One complaint regarding much that has been written about polyamory (both within the community and in mainstream media) is that its emphasis is often solely on sex. As a response to this, I try to focus on all aspects of polyamorous relationships, not just the fun, exciting, orgasmic ones.

When sex is given priority over other significant relationship issues, people's conceptions of polyamory are skewed. But it has another

negative effect as well: it overlooks an entire segment of poly relationships that has been nearly neglected in the current body of work on
the subject: committed relationships that do not include sex at all. In
fact, the respondents I spoke to for this book seemed to divide into two
camps: those who defined an important, intimate relationship as one
that includes a sexual component and those who had a broader vision
of what constitutes intimacy. In some nonsexual relationships, there
may be a certain amount of affection, flirting, sexual tension, erotic
touch, or romance, but there is no sex (however people define sex for
themselves). In others, there is no sexual relationship of any kind, yet
the participants consider themselves partners, even primary partners.
In her book *The Future of Love*, Daphne Rose Kingma discusses what
she calls "emotional spouses":

> An emotional spouse is a person with whom you share all
> your deep emotional intimacies, but with whom, for one
> reason or another, you choose not to be sexual. This may be
> because one or another partner in this relationship is gay, is
> married to someone else, is geographically unavailable, or
> shares none of the other aspects—daily life, or a shared
> household, for example—of a conventional relationship
> with you.[4]

Not all relationships have a sexual component. In some cases, a
relationship may have begun with a sexual element but the partners no
longer have sex. They are still very much committed to one another
and consider each other partners; the absence of sex does not change
that. For example, Alex and her partner have been together in a
polyamorous relationship for 11 years, even though they stopped
having sex several years ago. "We talked about the fact that she and
I weren't having sex. We weren't living in the same city. We both had
new people we were interested in and wanted different things," Alex
says. "I was more in Daddy mode at that point, that was part of who

I was at that time in my life. She wasn't interested anymore in that type of role, so we talked about it, and she said, 'It's not that I want to break up with you, or leave you, but the thing is, if you want to be in this relationship with me, we probably won't have sex ever again.'" They agreed to stay together and still consider each other primary partners.

Kathleen had a similar experience with her live-in partner, Guy. Over time, their sexual tastes changed, and it put a strain on their relationship:

> We realized that while we loved each other very much, it was very frustrating mentally and emotionally to try to make sex work. Some of the things that turn me on he has no interest in doing whatsoever. We had a lot of talks and we were really trying to push ourselves into making it work. When we finally said, Fuck it, let's take sex off the table, the relationship got better almost immediately. We didn't constantly feel as though we were failing the other person or we had to try to do something that wasn't comfortable for us. I was able to trust him again the way I had before I pulled back because I didn't know how to meet his needs. If we had been monogamous, we would have ended the relationship totally.

Many people I interviewed referred to a partner as a best friend—a relationship that was incredibly important, deeply intimate, and central to their lives but had no sexual component. Elizabeth, a 35-year-old attorney from Chicago, has a primary partner of four and a half years, and another partner Elizabeth calls her best friend. Although they once had a sexual relationship, they no longer do. "I would characterize my best friend as my 'secondary relationship' based on my emotional connection to her, my responsibility to her, my day-to-day time commitment to her. Whether we are having sex right now or not makes no difference to our emotional attachment. It just defines how we express that emotional attachment."

For some, a significant relationship has a specific or idiosyncratic dynamic that isn't encompassed by the prevailing types of relationships. Ruby Grace says, "I have a romantic but nonsexual relationship, but we don't have a word for it. We're very much in love with each other, care very much about each other, and it's our desire and intention to build a life together." Denise has a relationship based on mentoring and Dominance/submission: "Donna and I have been close friends for over five years now. I introduced her to the BDSM scene. There has never been any sexual tension between us; we're more like soul mate friends or even siblings in some ways... Our relationship is dynamic, compelling, and deeply intimate, it's simply not sexual or erotic. She holds the same degree of significance in my world as a romantic partner, you just need to replace the idea of romance with the idea of power exchange."

Nonsexual poly relationships can arise in all sorts of situations. In a recently documented phenomenon among gay and lesbian people, two couples or a couple and a single person join together to have children. For example, a lesbian couple ask a close gay male friend to donate sperm so they can have a child. If the man wants to play a role in the child's life, the three agree to be co-parents. He lives with them, helps raise the kid, and they all share a deep bond. In a mixed-orientation marriage, one spouse is straight and the other comes out as gay or lesbian. The spouses may stay together and consider themselves partners, but they no longer have a sexual relationship. They may become involved in sexual and loving relationships with others, but those are considered secondary to theirs.

Then there are multipartner relationships where not all partners are sexual with one another. For example, one woman is married to and sexually involved with two men. While the two men are not sexual with one another, they have a unique relationship that may encompass deep love, trust, and commitment. The two men may call each other partners, co-husbands, or co-spouses.

Nonsexual polyamory shows how polyamorous people have rejected another aspect of the prevailing view of relationships: that in order to have a significant other, one must have a sexual relationship. They have chosen instead to take a broader view of how partnerships and relationships can be defined based on their own beliefs, values, and experiences. As a result, people in poly relationships may be more likely to stay together: even when the sexual component of a relationship changes or ends, the relationship does not have to end. By redefining what constitutes an intimate relationship, partners can honor all the elements of their connection with each other.

PROFILE: LENA AND GAVIN

"We are committed to each other and never have forgotten where 'home' is."

LENA, 54, IS A LEGAL SECRETARY AND GAVIN, 43, is a project manager. They have been together for two years and consider each other primary partners.

When did you first start to explore polyamory?

Lena: I was actually a pretty mainstream person growing up, not a conservative person especially; nevertheless, I wouldn't call myself a radical of any kind. The first time you get a divorce, you think, Okay, I'll try again and we'll get it right and any guilt will be absolved and life will be good. But my second divorce hit me really hard. I grappled for a long time with the idea of a monogamous marriage because I could see how hard it was to be all things to one person over the long term. That had been a major issue in both of my marriages: whether we could really meet each other's needs. I was very skittish about getting emotionally involved with anyone for a long time... Once my daughter was about ready to exit high school, I felt it was okay to explore an interest I'd had for a long time: dating women... The second woman I dated said, "I need you to know that I have a husband." "Does he know that you're out with me?" I asked. "Oh yeah, he knows." Then she said, "I need you to know I also have a wife." I said, "Wow. Tell me more!" She took me home to meet them. We got into a real fun relationship for a while. That's when I was really enthusiastic about my bisexuality too, so I thought, What could be better than one of each? Plus I recognized the things that a poly relationship would offer me that a monogamous one wouldn't in terms of flexibility, and also honesty.

Gavin: My first wife and I were high school sweethearts. The sex was good prior to the marriage, and after that it kind of fizzled out. She suffers from depression, so her libido went down and we were in counseling many times to try to deal with it. One of the ways I dealt with it was I started going to massage parlors—I would get a massage and then get jacked off. I enjoyed it but after a while started to feel very guilty, especially when I became president of my church board. I told her about the massage parlors, and she ended our marriage. With my second wife, sex was really great in the beginning, and then things started going downhill. I had several affairs but felt guilty about cheating... I saw a Penn & Teller Show, *Bullshit*, and some HBO things about sex and various alternative communities, and I thought, I want that kind of life where it's open, it's honest, it's okay to have more than one partner.

Gavin, you mentioned church. What is your religion?

Gavin: I've been a Unitarian Universalist for a long time. I think UUs and poly people go together. The first principle is the inherent working dignity of all people. It's not just one person. If I think that somebody else is very worthy, I want to be able to express that and love that person just as much as this person. Justice, equity, and compassion in all human relations. Not just one person—all. I think it's important that we try to be friendly, certainly; if we can be loving to more than one person, that's okay. The never-ending search for truth and meaning. Well, for me, the truth is, monogamy doesn't work for me. I tried it, I've been dishonest with it, and it doesn't work for me.

Lena: The spirituality part of poly means being able to make a heart connection with more than one person and have that kind of emotional intimacy and the sharing of physical intimacy as well… To me, it is spiritually gratifying to know that I have the freedom to connect on that level with more than one person.

What's difficult about being polyamorous?

Lena: When you start talking about sharing partners, you raise some emotions that are very natural. Jealousy is something that we are going to feel. I've had jealous feelings with some of the relationships he's gotten into. I call it "getting the yips." I've been a little nervous, and he and I have done some processing about it. Once he goes out and has sex with them, it's all fine. It's the anticipation that's difficult. We don't know what's going to happen when we have a sexually intimate relationship with someone, especially if we're open to a heart connection as well. It's that unknown, what the future will bring, that makes me nervous.

Gavin: I am blessed to have someone who is so supportive, loving, and sexually open. I can live my authentic self because of her. She has transformed me. Although I occasionally date others, we are committed to each other and never have forgotten where "home" is.

Chapter 8

Solo Polyamory

IN AMERICAN CULTURE, monogamy isn't the only norm when it comes to relationships; it's expected that everyone wants to be and should be part of a couple. The fact of the matter is that some people prefer not to be in a partnered relationship—they just don't want a primary partner. They may like to live alone or, if they live with others, they don't want those others to be lovers. They are usually strongly independent. Although they enjoy relationships, they are content to have dates, lovers, friends, and partners, but don't consider anyone a primary partner. They may choose to devote the majority of their time and energy to education, parenting, spiritual pursuits, travel, or career. Having a primary relationship is not at the top of their priority list.

Some may call these folks single, but single has many different meanings and not all of them apply. When you check the "single" box on a legal form, it means you are not married—but you can be dating, in a committed relationship, or in a nonlegal marriage, as with two gay people. Single could mean you're dating, but not committed, or it could mean you're not dating at all. Rather than referring to them as single, I call these people solo polyamorists: they are dedicated to polyamory but they choose not to have a primary partner.

Solo polyamory can be temporary, time-limited, or long-term. Perhaps you just got out of a relationship, have decided to concentrate on yourself, and don't want to partner with anyone. Maybe you don't want a partner until your kids grow up and move out of the house; or you're in school and want to focus on your education for several years. Or you're currently dating and don't consider anyone you're seeing a partner, but if a relationship moved in that direction, that may change. Or you're just not interested in a primary relationship at all in the fore- seeable future. In general, people who practice solo polyamory date and have nonprimary partners, but they don't want to cohabit, mingle finances and resources, raise children, or make important life decisions with a partner.

After being in and out of relationships for 25 years, Nicole made a choice not to pursue a primary relationship: "I needed to become myself for a while. I've started my own company, and I'm doing my doctorate. Until that's done, I can't put the energy into a primary rela- tionship. That's of course saying that a primary relationship doesn't pop up and jump out at me between now and then. You can't stop it when it does. But I'm not looking."

Thomas's marriage ended four years ago, and he is not looking for a new significant other. He calls himself single and poly, though his relationship with one of his partners has grown deeper: "I've fallen in love and there is definitely a sense of things developing in that rela- tionship. We don't necessarily have rules that we have to follow or anything... I think it's like getting a date to the prom—I know who I'd ask, but fortunately, I don't need a date to the prom. I can go stag."

Solo polyamory may be your preference if:

- you like to have sex with different people, but prefer not to have a relationship with anyone
- you like to date, but can't see yourself dating one person exclusively

- you want relationships with multiple people—some of which may be serious or committed—but don't want a primary relationship or a primary partner
- you prefer to date and have sex and relationships with couples, but don't want to partner with them
- having a serious, committed, or primary relationship is not a priority in your life
- you enjoy freedom, independence, and solitude
- you aren't dating anyone currently, but if you were, it would be a polyamorous relationship

To do solo polyamory well, you should inform the people you date or have sex with that you have limited time and energy to devote to relationships. Many people assume that if they want a serious relationship, so does everyone else; you've got to confront those assumptions and be specific about what *you* want. When you make something other than your relationships your main priority, you also need to walk the walk. It can be easy to fall into seeing someone more than you want to out of habit or convenience. For Nicole, the biggest challenge of being solo and poly is not falling back into old patterns: "The challenge is not going and grabbing the first person that appears to be 'it'—grabbing onto them and getting all those security blankets hooked in again. Because usually at that point you're overlooking the issues that might also be wrapped in that blanket." Thomas would tell women he was dating right away that he was poly and bisexual. They would hear him, but still have other expectations; when he stuck to being poly, they'd often end the relationship because it hadn't progressed to a different level.

I consider myself to be my primary partner. This is a very real label for me, not something that I adopt while waiting for "The One" to come along. I am my own husband and wife. —Hailey

How and what you negotiate with someone will depend first and foremost on who else is in the picture. For example, the dynamic of two solo poly persons hooking up is much different from the dynamic of a solo person forming a relationship with someone who is partnered. In the case of the latter, the solo person may have to abide by the rules of her partner's primary relationship. Agreeing to someone else's limits may or may not work for you.

As with nonprimary partners in the previous chapter, the relationship choices you make as a solo polyamorous person are just as valid as those of people in primary relationships. While you may not have a serious commitment to any one partner, you still must negotiate the amount of time you spend together, safer sex, and other boundaries. Because your relationships may not be daily or time-intensive, you may feel disconnected from your partners; it may take some patience to reestablish your connection each time you get together. And, of course, being a nonprimary partner doesn't mean you are a second-class citizen: everyone deserves respect, compassion, and love. Adam says, "One thing that people most misunderstand about solo poly people is that the relationships we form are not shallow or disposable. I've been treated like shit by monogamous people who insist that I could only possibly see them as a fuck toy—and who treat me as one when it's not appropriate."

If you feel that your needs are not being met, you must speak up for yourself rather than chalking it up to your solo status. But you also need to be prepared, especially if you are dating someone who has a primary partner. If something big comes up in your partner's primary relationship—a new baby, a serious illness, or a major life change, for example—you may not get the time and attention you want, or any time and attention at all, for a period of time. Events such as these are not necessarily obstacles, but something to consider. Kathleen's partner is married and recently had a child: "If his wife is having a hard night, my play date gets canceled. Part of me is disappointed, but part of me is okay because one of the things I love about him is his commitment to his family."

An individual who is a primary partner to one person and a nonprimary partner to another has the opportunity to experience what both kinds of relationships have to offer, and they can fall back on one partner for support when something goes awry with the other. However, solos must consciously create a support system for themselves that is not partner-based. Again, the solo model flies in the face of our couples-centric culture, but there are plenty of people doing it *and* making it work.

Potential Issues and Conflicts in This Style

Triangles

If you are in a relationship with a partnered couple, you may feel that you have been put in the middle of an unhealthy dynamic. Sometimes, couples consciously or unconsciously use a third person as a buffer between them. Do not allow yourself to become an indirect communication device for a twosome, a constant conflict mediator, or a tool to make one partner jealous. If you find that each of them comes to you often to talk about the other, or you get contradictory information from them, consider it a warning that you've been sucked into a couple's drama. You can also feel that you have been put in the middle of a relationship even if you're only involved with one member of a couple—for example, if you spend a lot of time processing their other relationship. All relationships that share a partner are interconnected, and what happens in one can affect the others in many ways. As a solo, do not allow yourself to be put in the middle. Be clear with each of your partners about how you share information, focus on the relationship between just the two of you, and don't become part of any drama-filled love/lust triangles.

Societal Stigma

Because society assumes that you're either in a couple or actively look-ing to be in one, a solo person bucks the system; add your commit-ment to polyamory and you're double trouble. While suspicion of single bachelors and derision of old maids are no longer as prevalent as they were in the 20th century, adults who are not in a relationship are often discriminated against in both subtle and overt ways. Holidays, religious ceremonies, hotel and vacation packages, weddings, social events, restaurant seating, two-for-one deals—are all geared toward couples. Stereotypes about nonpartnered people abound: you're promiscuous; you're selfish and immature; you're emotionally challenged; you're afraid of intimacy and commitment; you're unwilling to "finally settle down." From movies to self-help books, the message is clear: there is something wrong with you if you are not part of a couple.

It's difficult for people constantly bombarded with these messages to go against the grain and do what works for them. Many solo people face insecurity, doubt, and self-judgment, all difficult to cope with when there is not a lot of support for their chosen relationship style. You have to tune out the endless propaganda and take pride in knowing who you are and what works for you.

> There's this part of me that's still dealing with that "as a woman you're not complete unless you have somebody" cultural thing. It takes a while to come face to face with the way you were raised and the unspoken stories you were told about what life was.
> —Kathleen

Lack of Community Support

Just as single people in society generally lack support and understand-ing, solo polyfolk are often underrepresented in writing about polyamory. Although people who practice open relationships challenge the myth of monogamy and redefine relationships, many community resources are aimed at people who want some kind of primary relationship. During my research, in fact, some solos criticized my interview questions for being geared toward partnered people. The culture of coupledom has seeped into our consciousness and become so pervasive that even people whose relationships challenge monogamy assume that most people want a primary relationship. Whether you choose to practice solo polyamory for a short time or as a dedicated lifestyle, it has its benefits and challenges, just like other styles of open relationships. Be prepared to forge your own path as you shatter myths not only about monogamy, but also about couplehood.

PROFILE: NICOLE

*"Each relationship has a very sexual component,
so when we can get together it's a sexual thrill."*

NICOLE IS A 46-YEAR-OLD BISEXUAL WOMAN, a self-employed consultant currently pursuing her PhD, who lives in northern Virginia. Nicole's first marriage lasted only six months. She was married to her second husband for 20 years; they have two children together, 14 and 17. When her second marriage ended, she did some serious soul searching: "When I sat down and analyzed all my relationships, even from high school, I [realized that I] always got in trouble with whomever I was dating because I would be friends with other men. I would think of the other men as my buddies—it wasn't like I was sleeping with them or anything. But the person I was dating was always jealous, jealous, jealous." Yet her jealous boyfriends would end up cheating on her.

After years of unsatisfying monogamy, she decided she wanted a change. Four years ago, she got involved with a divorced man: "We actually sat down early in our relationship and brainstormed the ideal relationship style. We had no idea what polyamory was, we had no idea what swinging was. We decided that we would start out with what was traditionally considered a swinging relationship. Then, as we got more comfortable, [we'd] work our way into more of a poly type [of relationship]. We dreamed all this up and said, 'We've figured this out, let's go about it.' Well, unfortunately I went about it the way we'd agreed, but he did not. It took me about four years to see that he was using poly as a front for cheating."

Today, she identifies herself as polyamorous and currently has relationships with six people; the newest one has been going on for only two months, and the oldest for two and a half years. "I've started each relationship by having a chat with the [person's] primary, to say, I'm not here to steal your man. I just want to have a friend, an intimate friend… I just want a community I can be with, I can have dinner with, I can talk to without having to hide what it is I do. I want family, I want friends, I want lovers. I don't want a husband. I don't want to take him away from you. Right now, my relationships are working wonderfully. I think this is because we have no demands on each other. We enjoy the time we have together, and we get together when time allows. I respect their primary relationships, and they don't get possessive or upset about any of my relationships. Each of the relationships has a very sexual component, so when we can get together it's a sexual thrill."

For Nicole, the only downside is feeling lonely at times without a daily companion: "I don't have anyone to sleep with every night or cry on their shoulder or tell the joys of the day, and that's really a lot of human bonding. I'm used to having that and I don't have it right now, and that's tough. I do get that bonding when I can get my secondary partner's ear for a little bit. But I don't want to be whiny and moany. I want support, but I don't want them to think I'm needy. They have their own primaries, so they get all of that stuff from them."

Chapter 9

Polyfidelity

THE TERM *POLYFIDELITY* was coined to describe the relationship structure of the Kerista Commune, a San Francisco community with between six and 30 members during its 20-year existence from 1971 to 1991. Modern polyfidelity describes a multipartner group of three or more people who have made a commitment to each other to be in a primary relationship. Although the number of partners varies, the most common polyfidelitous relationships have three, four, or five partners—a group rarely has more than six. Groups larger than that usually consider themselves a family, tribe, or network whose members are interrelated but do not form a single relationship unit.

You might choose polyfidelity if:

- you want multiple intimate and significant relationships and have the capacity to love more than one person at a time
- you have several partners who want to form a committed group
- you're part of a couple and want to form a committed relationship with one or more others or another couple
- you are committed to the members of a relationship unit and have no desire for relationships outside the unit

- you are committed to the members of a relationship unit but you also desire relationships outside the unit

Polyfidelitous groups often, but not always, live together, and they may do things that many committed couples do: they are fluid-bonded, make important decisions together, share resources, raise children, and otherwise behave as a family unit. All of the members are committed to each other and to the group as their primary relationship.

Owen and Carlie were together for two and a half years when Carlie discovered she was bisexual and wanted to explore her attraction to women. Owen was supportive: "At first, we just thought we'd be swingers because we didn't have any intention of having another primary partner. We hadn't even thought about that." They met and began a sexual relationship with Alexis, which turned into something deeper. Alexis, their triad partner of two years, says, "I never expected this. I don't even really consider myself to be polyamorous. I just happened to fall in love with a couple."

Ivan, Turner, and Lewis, three gay men, live together as a triad in upstate New York. Turner and Lewis were in a nonmonogamous relationship for nine years, and they have been with Ivan for over a year. Turner says: "I consider there to be four distinct relationships: 1) me and Ivan, 2) me and Lewis, 3) Ivan and Lewis, and 4) the three of us. If I had to identify one as primary, it would be the 'trilationship' between the three of us because our interdependence guides our approach, decisions and success." The most difficult part for Ivan is telling other people: "It's a challenge to explain our life to others. Sometimes this is a matter of career safety and sometimes it is more of a lack of understanding of *what* we are. Many assume that we're 'two plus one' or a 'couple and their boy'—not the three equals sharing one life and one bed that we are."

In a triad such as Ivan's, all members have a sexual relationship with each other. In other polyfidelitous groups, some members may

not have sex or a romantic relationship with all other members—
for example, in a V triad where a woman has two husbands or a man
has two wives. However, the two "tips" of a V triad often consider
themselves significant others and co-spouses.

Some larger multipartner groups are made up of a combination of
preexisting couples and singles. The bigger a group becomes, the less
likely it is they all cohabit. Usually, not all members of a large multipartner group are sexual with each other, and each person may have a
different level of connection and intimacy with other members of the
group.

Brett is a 72-year-old retired aerospace engineer from California
who teaches college. He is part of a five-person W that includes his
wife, Vicki, his wife's partner/his co-husband Mark, Mark's wife, Mary,
and Mary's partner Ross. Brett describes the genesis of the W: "We
had known Mark and Mary for several years, professionally and per-
sonally, through the Unitarian Universalist church and the university.
Mary asked my wife one day about open relationships and the gals
had a lunch talk. We were invited for dinner, and I told my wife that
I expected the evening to be fun, but she doubted me. I was right—
we all played together in the hot tub and the bedroom. My wife and
Mark became deeply enmeshed immediately; she had known and
liked him for years, so this was a perfect relationship for them. They
are matched in sex drive and many other interests. He has become my
best male friend. Mary immediately told Ross, a friend of hers, she
was no longer monogamous, and they became lovers. Over the seven
years, we have become one lovely family, sharing beds, dinners, vacation time-shares, cars, and lovers." The five don't live together but
they spend a significant amount of time together: "My wife is clearly
primary, we share lives fully, live together, share all financial assets,
etc. I call her my custodial spouse," Brett says. "Mark spends three
nights a week in our bed and four nights at his home with Mary." The
five are fluid-bonded with each other, but rarely all have sex together.

Benefits of Polyfidelity

There are many benefits of multipartner poly groups. Being involved with more than one partner gives members more ways to express themselves and have their needs met. This leads to greater satisfaction and fulfillment in their relationships. "We all have strengths and weaknesses, and we can work collaboratively to reinforce once another. Additionally, it provides 'built in' variety sexually," Ivan says.

If all partners live together, they can draw on multiple incomes to share expenses and resources; they also have more help with the basic chores of life like household duties and childcare. Emma is in a triad with a man and a woman: "My husband works full-time and is the main breadwinner. My wife works part-time and then throws pots part time while she tries to get her pottery business off the ground. I am a housewife. While they are out of the house, I do all of the cleaning and shopping. This frees up our collective time together. We have more free time than any of our other friends who are in traditional relationships."

More partners also means more physical and emotional support, which is especially significant during major life changes or times of crisis. For example, Leslie was diagnosed with breast cancer shortly after one husband, Ed, moved in with her and her other husband, Colin. Having both men to take care of her was a blessing for everyone: "Ed told me that he would not want to be my only husband."

Sandra is a 43-year-old massage therapist from the Pacific Northwest. Her five-person poly circle is made up of herself, her husband, Rick, her male partner Doug, Doug's wife, Gabrielle, and Sandra and Rick's girlfriend Joan. Sandra, Rick, Doug, and Gabrielle live and raise their four children together in a house they own jointly. Joan lives on the East Coast; she talks to the others on the phone every day and sees them every two months; she has a sexual relationship with only Sandra and Rick. While each member of the circle is not sexual with every other member, they are all committed to each other for the long haul.

Sandra recalls a time when their circle particularly worked well: "Recently Doug's mom died. Gabrielle was scheduled to have surgery on the date of the funeral. Gabrielle asked me to attend the funeral with Doug and their children, while Rick stayed home to care for Gabrielle and our children. Joan felt represented by me in the company of Doug's extended family, who welcomed me as an important member of Doug's immediate family. It seems very logistical, but the comfort and emotional support that we all felt in this difficult time was beyond what the usual 'friends' could offer." (For more on this circle of five, see the profile at the end of Chapter 17, Raising Children.)

Polyfidelitous Configurations

triad: three people who all have sexual and love relationships with each other

V triad: a unit of three in which two of the members are not romantic/sexual with each other [1]

quad: a unit of four. The most common configurations are:

1) two male/female couples where the women are sexual with both men but not with each other, and the men are sexual with both women but not with each other;

2) two male/female couples where the women are sexual with both men and with each other, and the men are sexual only with both women;

3) four people of any gender who are all sexual with each other

poly circle, poly family, W, or pod: [2] groups of five or more

W: a fivesome (think of it as two connected V's)

Negotiation and Potential Issues

Open versus Closed

Some polyfidelitous groups are closed, meaning that all partners are monogamous within the group. Sandra's five-person circle is closed to outside partners; four of the five own a house and raise children together. All the members, including the one who doesn't live with them, have agreed that they have sex only with each other.

In an open polyfidelitous group, members may have additional partners. If the group is open to sex or BDSM partners, they practice something similar to partnered nonmonogamy, with a group at the center instead of a couple. For example, the triad of Carlie, Alexis, and Owen has agreed that if one member wants to be sexual with nontriad members, all three have to be present; they may or may not also be involved. In Diane's triad, "Rules about playing outside the triad are pretty simple. All one has to do is ask permission to be with someone, and it is usually given. If it isn't, there is usually a damn good reason why not, like the person being skanky or unsafe, or has had personal problems in the past."

If the group is open to additional relationships, it is simply another form of polyamory—in most cases, the group is primary and other significant relationships are secondary. Leslie is a 36-year-old housewife from Minneapolis. She married Colin, a computer programmer, 12 years ago. Six years ago, she became involved with Ed. The three now live together in a V triad and she considers both men her husbands: "We are lifemated. I am legally married to one and would be to the other if it was legal." They have agreed they can have other partners outside the triad, as long as they practice safer sex with them. They are even open to an additional primary partner, but that would take lots of negotiation. Colin admits that the emotional part of relationships outside the triad is sometimes difficult for him: "[The hardest thing is] being clear in my own mind about how far I can go with

someone emotionally, and how much of myself I can give to a relationship when I have a marriage I'm committed to. I have a tendency to
just want to get more and more intimate with people."

Emma, Penny, and George have been a closed triad for several
years, and they recently renegotiated to become open to outside relationships. "One of the things that have come up is that we are not trying
to open up just so that we can have sex for the sake of sex," Emma
says. "I feel very strongly that the potential lover needs to be someone
I have a connection with. Does it have to be love? No. But it does need
to be more than just fucking. At least for me, presently; I believe the
other two agree. If this openly poly thing doesn't work out because of
other people's inability to do it, then my marriage will come before my
desire to become more openly poly."

Shawn says, "To quote a friend, my life is fairly normal once you
get over the fact that I have a wife and a girlfriend. I can't possibly contemplate the idea of starting a relationship with someone they didn't
approve of, because any time I spend with the other person is time I'm
taking away from them. So they have to agree that it's worth it to them
to lose that time for me to spend it with a third person. I love them.
I'm planning on spending the rest of my life with them. I want them
happy."

Communication and Logistics

One of the benefits of having more than one partner is that there's more
than one person to call you on your shit. In his book *Pagan Polyamory*,
Raven Kaldera calls couples "the most stable form of relationship and
also the most prone to stagnation, rigidity, and self-delusion."[3]
Members of a couple can grow quite comfortable with the dysfunctional patterns of their dynamic—there's no one around to say, "I
notice that you avoid this topic whenever it comes up." When another
person enters the mix, it can really shake things up. In their book *Group
Marriage,* Larry and Joan Constantine write about marriage partners'

repeated behavior patterns (the script) and the unspoken agreements (the contract) they make to play certain roles. The Constantines posit that a multiperson marriage exposes these elements:

> Repeatedly we found that the intense, intimate, open environment of the multilateral marriage exposed the scripts and the terms of the contract to the couples involved. The new context made old behaviors stand out in sharp contrast; habituated responses are difficult to see while situations remain unchanged.[4]

When one person tells you something about yourself, you can ignore it more easily—you can think it is just their opinion or chalk it up to misperception. But when two people who know you well tell you something, it's much harder to ignore, especially when it's not a friend or acquaintance looking at the relationship from the outside, but someone *in* the relationship—who has deep, intimate knowledge of the players, personalities, and dynamics. This level of intimacy coupled with accountability can help members of polyfidelitous relationships change and grow.

The other side of that coin, though, is this: the more people in a relationship, the more difficult communication can become. Every member must work to stay connected to the others, so no one feels left out of the loop. In a polyfidelitous relationship, there are more people to process feelings with, more people's needs and desires to consider, and often more decisions to make. Plus, since all members are committed to each other, everyone must have a voice in decision making. If the group is open to outside partners, everyone needs to negotiate and agree on the boundaries for those relationships.

We try very hard to keep communication open, although, in a marriage of three, it is hard to keep track of who we have told and who we haven't. Besides, we joke that people who are married never talk, so there are plenty of times when one or two of us know something and the third doesn't. —Emma

When three or more partners are involved, the basics of daily life must be negotiated to make room for everyone in the relationship, whether it's who sleeps with whom and when, whose parents you visit for the holidays, or how you handle work and vacation schedules. Whether or not everyone lives under the same roof, you need to make the time to nurture and cultivate each relationship as well as have time for yourself. This balancing of time and energy is an issue faced by most people in nonmonogamous relationships, but it is especially important when you have multiple primary relationships.

Co-spouse Relationships

In his book *Pagan Polyamory*, Raven Kaldera cautions people about one of the less constructive dynamics that can develop in a V (or what I call a V triad):

> Being at the point of a V is the hardest role in polyamory because it means you have two people's full-time attention and needs focused on you. It means that you may be expected to mediate between them, and perhaps less focus is placed on their ability to communicate, because of course you're there, and you've learned to speak both their languages, and since they're both there for you, why should they bother to have much of a relationship with each other?[5]

Kaldera's quote raises the issue of the nature of the relationship between co-spouses in a V triad or in another group in which all members do not have a sexual or romantic relationship. There are few models for how to develop communication, trust, even emotional intimacy with a person who is both your significant other's significant other *and* someone you've committed to share your life with as well. Daria and Audrey are in a V triad with Shawn; about her relationship with Audrey, Daria says, "We're family, certainly. Any life choices that either of us makes are definitely going to affect the other. We live together, we're planning to grow old together. Our relationships are so entwined, she is definitely my partner as well, regardless of any romantic intent."

It was the Hawaiian custom at one time to permit men and women to have more than one mate. A man's wives or a woman's husbands are punalua *to each other. The term is also used to refer to the relationship between two people who share a longtime lover, regardless of marital status, or between a person's former and current mate.*

—PLURAL LOVES: DESIGNS FOR BI AND POLY LIVING[6]

"We're very good friends who are in a relationship, just without the sex," Audrey adds. In general, women in these relationships seem to have an easier time than men being close, nonsexual partners.

Two straight men in a V triad are in uncharted territory, since most men are not encouraged by society to bond with other men intimately. For example, to outward appearances, Timothy, Meredith, and William are in a V triad: Meredith is in a relationship with both Timothy and William, and they all live together (though this is a new development in the last few months). They don't see themselves as a committed, cohesive unit. The men call each other friends but do not consider themselves co-spouses or co-boyfriends; their relationship with each other is tenuous at best—they tolerate each other. As with most kinds of nontraditional relationships, the dynamics of intimacy between straight men in a triad are up for interpretation and negotiation, and they change over time.

Colin and Ed are in a V triad with Leslie; though they consider each other co-husbands, theirs is a relationship that our culture doesn't really have a name for. Ed says:

In the past, I have described my relationship with Colin as like a relationship with a brother. We don't tease each other like I see most brothers do, and we are much more comfortable being naked and expressing sexual thoughts about Leslie to each other. While I was working and going to school several years ago, it was his suggestion that he and Leslie pay for my housing and food, and give me a stipend, which was a bit of a shock to me. He is generous in a way that is different from the way that I am, and it is surprising sometimes. I expect that we would continue to live together for some time if we outlive Leslie, and I think the flavor of our relationship is something like family members that share the same ideology and outlook on life. Colin is like family I never had.

Odd One Out

Groups of three or more can create complex power dynamics; for example, you should be conscious of not ganging up on one partner or allowing one to feel left out. This can be especially true in a triad, where one person may easily feel excluded or less valued. In a triad one person may also feel caught in the middle, having to play mediator between the other two. It could be that two people have a more forceful arguing style and the third doesn't always feel his or her voice is heard. Emma, who calls her triad partners "spice" (the plural of spouse), says, "It is difficult anytime one of my spice comes to rely on me completely, essentially shutting the other person out. If there is some sort of rift or fight between the two of them, they come to me for support, to feel better, and to bitch. Feeling like the fulcrum in the middle is the worst part about a triad."

Shawn is involved with Daria and Audrey in a V triad. Before Daria, Shawn and Audrey agreed that they could do anything "up to penetration with a penis" with other partners. When Daria entered the picture, she wasn't comfortable with that agreement, so Shawn agreed to limit his sexual activities to "making out and fondling" only. Shawn says, "You play to the level of the least comfortable person, if you want to keep everybody happy."

Relationship Recognition

While the members of many triads, quads, and other polyfidelitous groups consider themselves all married to each other, legally they are not. In fact, in the majority of the triads I interviewed, two members are legally married. In some cases, they held a separate ceremony to acknowledge and celebrate the third member and the triad. When Owen and Carlie got married, their triad partner, Alexis, was the maid of honor. The night before the wedding, the three held a ceremony with Alexis's parents in which Owen and Carlie presented Alexis with a ring. "Owen and I thought it was really important to demonstrate our commitment to her parents, especially since they were coming to the wedding," Carlie says. "I wanted to demonstrate that I'm serious about Alexis and it's not just a phase I'm going through. I'm not just getting married and having someone on the side. I'm really committed to Alexis. I love Alexis and take this very seriously. I didn't want her family to think otherwise."

A ceremony such as this is an important ritual for honoring partners' commitment to each other; however, their relationship is not legally recognized or rewarded. One partner (or more) in a polyfidelitous relationship is often left without health care benefits, spousal rights, or custody of children. George says, "Society isn't set up for us, so things like medical benefits and legal partner rights that don't extend to a third person make things difficult. We still have to deal with making provisions for Penny having legal rights to the kids, if, god forbid, something were to happen to Emma and me." Polyfidelitous partners must create legal agreements to protect certain aspects of their relationships. (For more on this subject, see Chapter 19, Legal and Practical Issues.)

In addition to lacking legal recognition, often a polyfidelitous group is not recognized by parents, friends, or the community. Sometimes, two people in a triad or one couple in a fivesome are acknowledged and others are thought to be friends or housemates. This can be stressful, alienating, and difficult. For more on dealing with the outside world, see Chapter 16, Coming Out (or Not), Finding Community, Creating Families.

PROFILE: LEWIS, TURNER, AND IVAN

"We consider ourselves a 'trilationship' with three equal sides."

LEWIS, 50, TURNER, 37, AND IVAN, 37, are white, well-educated gay men. One works in telecommunications, one works for the government, and one is a professor; they are all active in political organizations. They live together as a triad in upstate New York.

Lewis and Turner first connected during an anonymous erotic encounter at an adult bookstore; several years later, they met again and began dating. They have been together for 10 years. Their relationship was monogamous at first, though they were open to lots of flirting with other men. Eventually, they began having casual sex with others (always as a couple). At around the eight-year mark, both had been traveling separately a lot for work and they agreed that each could hook up with others on his own.

About a year and a half ago, Turner attended a conference where he met Ivan. The two connected immediately. When Turner came home, he told Lewis about Ivan. "I said to Lewis—and this is the first time I ever used these words—'Something about my emotional connection to Ivan makes me feel like I'm cheating. I don't know what this means, but I don't want to lose Ivan as a part of my life.' Lewis's first reaction was: tricks and fun with other people was one thing, but having an important relationship on the side was not going to happen. That was not part of our makeup, that was not part of where we were." The concept of a poly relationship was completely new to Ivan, and he wasn't sure about it. Turner asked Lewis to start communicating with Ivan to get to know him. Lewis agreed, and he and Ivan began communicating by telephone, via email, and in virtual face-to-face sessions with a webcam; they began to really like each other.

Lewis told Ivan that he was starting to develop strong feelings for him. He said, "Because I am enough years older than you and Turner, I expect you to be around to take care of Turner when I'm gone." Ivan replied, "What makes you think that you're going to go first? It could be you and I." Lewis says, "He said it in such a way that I knew he meant that it didn't matter to him which one of us he ended up with, because he was learning to make a commitment to both of us as we were willing to make a commitment to him." He adds, with sarcasm, "So that's when I realized that he was worthy of my love."

About that time, Lewis and Turner confessed to a friend that they had a boyfriend. Lewis and Ivan still had not met. "That's just another piece of unconventionality that the rest of the world never really gets. How can you develop feelings for someone that you've never physically met? But we were spending, on some evenings and on weekends, six and seven hours talking to each other," Turner says. The next month, Ivan came to visit. He and Lewis hit it off. They immediately discussed the possibility of Ivan moving to New York from Iowa. Lewis and Turner began to tell their friends, who assumed the arrangement was all about having lots of sex.

The trio realized that they wanted to be clear with each other and other people that they were three equal partners, not Lewis and Turner and their plaything. They continued to date for a year as Ivan began applying for jobs in New York. When he was offered a position, he moved east to live with Lewis and Turner.

"I think that one of my biggest mistakes when Ivan first moved here was trying to micromanage the relationship [between him and Lewis]," Turner says. "Even though for a year it was fine...I think subconsciously I felt I needed to hold it together. That has more to do with my neurosis and my family background." In addition to the hardship of relocating, Ivan must deal with being the new guy, since Turner and Lewis are such an established couple in their community. When Turner explained it to his mom, "She went through a period of worrying whether this was a threat to my relationship with Lewis; she just didn't understand it. I tried the whole intellectual route. I told her, 'Honestly, everyone loves more than one person and people often lie about that. We're just not lying about it'... She moved from 'I don't really understand' to 'Okay, I'm putting him on the Christmas list. What does he want?'"

Chapter 10

Monogamous/ Nonmonogamous and Mono/Poly Combinations

A COUPLE MAY CHOOSE to adopt a hybrid style of open relationship, in which one partner is monogamous and the other is nonmonogamous. This occurs more often than you might think, yet it is one of the least talked about and most misunderstood styles. A mono/nonmono or mono/poly combination style could be as straightforward as a monogamous person getting into a relationship with a nonmonogamous one, where both partners know from the beginning that one wants additional partners and the other doesn't. Some relationships begin with both partners monogamous or both nonmonogamous and transform into a combo when the desires and needs of one partner change. As in other kinds of nonmonogamy, a significant difference between partners sometimes needs to be addressed; in this style, one partner is content to remain monogamous while the other has additional partners for sex, relationships, or both.

I know a female couple, Jane and Dory, who were together for 10 years. About a year into the relationship, Jane discovered she was interested in BDSM, but Dory was not. After lots of discussion, Dory told Jane she could explore BDSM with other people. Jane became involved with a woman who lived in a different state who became her Daddy, and they saw each other about every six weeks. Jane explained to me that BDSM was something she needed and it was very important, but it was the only area where she and Dory were incompatible. It wasn't something she wanted to lose Dory over. Jane got what she needed by spending intermittent weekends with her Daddy, but her primary commitment was to Dory.

A difference in sex drives is a common source of conflict in couples and one that can break up a relationship; however, it can also be an opportunity to shift one's expectations and negotiate a structure that works for both partners. If a low-libido partner meets the majority of the needs within the relationship except the sexual ones, a high-libido partner can seek sex outside the relationship to fulfill those needs. Similarly, celibacy can be a temporary or long-term choice in response to specific circumstances, such as serious physical or mental illness, injury, or depression, or simply as a personal choice. Many couples remain together even when both partners lose interest in sex. Unlike many therapists, self-help books, and even poly advocates, I believe that a relationship doesn't *need* to have an ongoing sexual component for it to be significant, committed, and viable. But what happens when one partner wants to remain sexual and the other doesn't? If one partner chooses celibacy and the other does not, then they can negotiate a combo style.

Hannah and Chiyo's mutual desire for BDSM and nonmonogamy brought them together. After nearly seven years, Hannah's interest in BDSM began to wane. She got more serious about martial arts, which consumed more of her time and filled her need for some of the intense physical activity she got from BDSM. In addition, she began experiencing menopause and she says her sex drive "went in the toilet." Gradually, she and Chiyo began to have discussions about their changing needs and desires, which led them to negotiate a mono/poly combination style with a few rules: no kissing other people, no sexual play with anyone else in their bedroom, safer sex, and Hannah would have veto power over potential new partners. They still have sex occasionally, but Chiyo's primary sexual relationships are with her two other partners, who are her Dominants.

"Hannah knows that I love her deeply and am committed to her. She also knows that I need, and I'm devoted to, my D/s relationships," Chiyo says. Hannah says she rarely gets jealous: "Our relationship is so strong that we've defined our primary relationship together and we feel so comfortable with each other. It's been that way all along. We've said all along we're primary to each other and nothing gets in the way of that... We've respected that this whole time and never lied to each other about anything. So I feel okay with it. At times I've grown jealous of the amount of time she spends with these people, but we work through that." She believes that trust is the key to their open relationship: "If you have doubts about what your partner is doing, then it'll never feel safe."

When one member of a heterosexual married couple comes out as gay or lesbian and the spouses stay together, they may or may not continue to be sexual. Some mixed-orientation spouses agree that the gay/lesbian spouse can pursue sex or relationships with same-gender partners while the straight spouse remains monogamous.

This style can work for you if:

- one partner wants sex with others, and the other doesn't
- one partner wants additional partners, and the other doesn't
- you want to accommodate some sexual difference or incompatibility by opening up the relationship, but one partner is content to remain monogamous

Examples of mono/nonmono combos

Bisexual and not bisexual: the bisexual partner has sexual or relationship partners of a different gender than the primary partner

Straight and gay/lesbian: the gay or lesbian partner has same-gender partners

Disabled and not disabled: the nondisabled partner explores sex or BDSM that the disabled partner has no interest in or cannot engage in as a result of the disability

Low libido and high libido: the partner with the high libido has additional sex partners

Kinky and nonkinky: the kinky partner has other partners specifically for BDSM play

Sexual and celibate: the sexual partner pursues sex with other people

Consent and Agreement

Consent is a crucial component of open relationships and must be made especially clear in monogamous/nonmonogamous combinations. The mono/nonmono structure is *not* a case of one partner getting "more" than the other, as it may appear on the surface. The monogamous partner should never feel pressured or coerced to accept the nonmonogamous partner's terms. Nor should she agree to this style out of fear of being rejected or abandoned. It can only work if the monogamous partner truly has no interest in additional sex or relationships—there is no place for martyrs in any kind of nonmonogamy. If a couple chooses this style to address some issue of incompatibility in the relationship, it must be approached as a solution that works for *both* partners. There must be a dialogue where both partners have input about the limits, boundaries, and rules. Both people—but especially the monogamous partner—need to be clear and confident about the relationship choice and must see it *as a choice*.

As with all kinds of open relationships, mono/poly and mono/nonmono relationships require agreements between the partners as well as a commitment to the relationship. The connection between the two of you—emotional, romantic, affectionate, sexual—must be nurtured as you embark on this new style. Likewise, your commitment to one another must be articulated, reinforced, honored, and respected.

As part of your negotiation, you should make an agreement about rules. For example, Coraline has two boyfriends, five lovers, and two BDSM play partners. One partner, Tom, is monogamous with her. So there are some rules with him: "We don't have sex if I've had sex with someone else in the past 24 hours. I don't have anal sex with anyone but him." Lynn has a less specific agreement with her monogamous partner: "I don't tell my girlfriend about the details of my interactions with other people unless she asks, and in return she doesn't expect that I set boundaries as to what I do with other people aside from expecting that I use common sense to ensure my safety, in both a physical and an emotional sense."

Potential Issues and Conflicts

Guilt

One potential issue for the nonmonogamous partner in this style is feeling guilty. Barbara has been with her partner for seven years; their relationship began as polyamorous, but for the past year and a half her partner has chosen to be monogamous. Barbara says, "About 10 months ago, I decided that I was no longer scared of monogamy, and didn't believe that it would 'make me crazy.' I embarked on a six-month commitment to monogamy... I decided that, while monogamy was nothing to fear, I didn't like it much, either." After her experiment with monogamy, Barbara returned to being polyamorous, but felt some guilt, which she had to deal with. "I had quite a lot of fear... The way I've been able to grapple with that is to say, well, I have to figure out what I want and then decide how to approach doing that. [I have to be] really careful not to just limit my own imagination and my own possibilities because somebody else is making a choice. They're making it for good reasons and for healthy reasons that I really support. My support doesn't mean giving up myself. I think a lot of people do that in relationships. They give up things that nobody asks them to give up; they just do it because it seems that's what you're supposed to do."

I think women who are nonmonogamous with a monogamous partner particularly struggle with guilt because they're unsure of themselves, feel as if they don't "deserve" to get everything they want, or believe they are somehow getting "more" than their monogamous partners. If you feel guilty about your choices, remember that your partner has agreed to them and the point is that the style works for both of you.

Resentment and Jealousy

Jealousy and resentment can occur in any relationship; in situations where both partners are nonmonogamous, these feelings can be mitigated by the fact that both people have other partners and get to experience both sides of jealousy. In a style where both partners are nonmonogamous, if you feel jealous that your partner is out of town with his other partner for the weekend, you know how he must have felt when you went on a trip for three days with your friend with benefits. In a mono/nonmono combo, jealous feelings can be lopsided. In these cases, both partners need to work on them. The monogamous partner should work on feeling secure, appreciate solitude, and have a solid support system. The nonmonogamous partner should make time for his partner and take care to reassure her.

Societal Stigma and Lack of Support

Gaining the support of your loved ones is an issue all people in open relationships must deal with. However, it can be especially tricky for people who practice a hybrid style. First, even someone who is supportive of open relationships may not understand this particular style. If you say, "My partner and I are exploring sex with other people," supportive folks may get the general concept. But if you say, "My partner is having sex [or relationships] with other people and I am not," you're liable to get a few raised eyebrows. Many people believe strongly that relationships should strive for equality, everyone giving and getting equal amounts of time, love, and attention. If this is the prevailing ideal, people cannot fathom how mono/poly could ever be fulfilling. It's the "You can't have your cake and eat it too" mentality. Even within polyamorous communities, some people see a monogamous/non-monogamous pairing as inherently unfair.

Mono/nonmono combos are criticized on several fronts. Here is some of the criticism you may hear: The monogamous person is being taken advantage of, used, and abused. The nonmonogamous person wouldn't be doing this if she really loved the monogamous person. Monogamous people and nonmonogamous people are too fundamentally different to have a relationship; you should have the same values and ideas about relationships, otherwise it's a deal breaker. This is just like polygamy, where a husband has multiple wives but a wife only has one husband—it's sexist, patriarchal, and coercive. It's not fair.

Barbara faced criticism from others as well as her internalized self-judgment: "One thing that I really enjoyed about poly was that it was very egalitarian... Now it feels a little bit like I question myself, what's given to me, and think that I now owe somebody. It's really fighting off those cultural assumptions. When somebody would ask me, 'What is this polyamory?' I'd be able to explain it. Then they would ask, 'Well, what about your boyfriend?' I'd say, 'Oh, he's not doing that [he's monogamous].' Then come the reactions: 'Well, why are you? What's wrong with you? What is it about you that you can't have a similar relationship?' I've been surprised to have those negative things creep in."

People negotiate and structure their relationships in unique ways. No one who is outside a relationship can judge what works inside it; we shouldn't invalidate other people's choices simply because they look different from our own. Open relationships are ultimately about choosing a relationship style that meets our needs; all styles are valid and valuable. If this style works for you, embrace it.

PROFILE: VIOLET AND RON

> *"I'd much rather have a happy, fulfilled lover than a frustrated, resentful one."*

RON, A 57-YEAR-OLD POLYAMOROUS MAN, is in a relationship with 49-year-old Violet, who is monogamous. They live in New York City, consider themselves "naturally introverted people," and have been partners for almost 10 years.

When Ron told Violet soon after they met that he was polyamorous, her first reaction was: "I meet this really interesting guy and now I can't go out with him because he won't be monogamous." While Violet understood the concept, she didn't have an interest in exploring polyamory herself: "For me having a significant relationship takes so much energy and time that I don't know how he does it. I need a lot of time to myself." They discussed it further, and she realized that "this makes a lot of sense and even though it's not for me, I liked him enough to want to keep going with it even though I was really scared. I didn't know how I would handle feelings of jealousy."

They agreed that he would maintain his current relationships but not seek out any new ones for a period of time. At first, Violet didn't want to know any details about his other relationships. Ron thought this was like lying by omission; it had an air of dishonesty and cheating. About four years into the relationship, Violet became more comfortable with hearing more about his other partners: "I know that [Ron wasn't] happy with the 'don't ask/don't tell,' but I needed it at the time; it worked for me. And we've evolved beyond that."

Violet had a big breakthrough after meeting one of Ron's other partners, Sherry. Sherry insisted that she meet Violet to make sure Violet consented to Ron having other partners. "She let me know that it was okay to feel triggered by things. There was one incident where I was triggered and I didn't think I could tell [Ron]... I always thought, Oh, I made this agreement now, so I have to bear everything. And she let me know that even poly people get jealous." Being allowed to feel jealous relieved a huge burden for Violet: "I need to be constantly vigilant to head off feelings of insecurity and jealousy. But this has the positive effect of forcing me to be in touch with how I feel, which has always been a problem for me... As I've become more secure in this relationship, feelings of jealousy have become nearly nonexistent."

Both tell a story about how their communication has deepened over the years. They had spent the night together and Ron was leaving to see his other partner. Violet said to him, "I haven't had enough of you this weekend." She says, "It took me a while to realize I could say things like that to him and not have him take it as, Oh, she wants me to stay, or something like that." For Ron, it was an important moment: "She wasn't trying to get me to stay, she wasn't trying to make me feel better, it was just a statement. And I remember how good I felt at the time... It wasn't that I needed Violet to have more, it was just that it was such a clean way of expressing what was the truth."

"Being poly makes it easier for me to have all sorts of relationships, sexual or otherwise, because there is no predetermined limit on any relationship I might have," Ron says. Violet concurs. "We are both very autonomous people, and his polyamory gives me a feeling of freedom. Plus, it makes my lover happy, and I'd much rather have a happy, fulfilled lover than a frustrated, resentful one." She says the most difficult thing is explaining their relationship to other people. "It just takes too much energy to explain to people so they'll understand that I'm not being used, abused, or cheated on." Ron adds: "In every relationship I had before, [as soon as it began] I was looking for the exits. But in Violet's case I'm not looking for the exits—probably because [she's] not blocking them." Violet says Ron gives her the one thing she needs most, which, until she met him, she believed could only come with monogamy: "My partner is very aware that I need to feel that I'm special to him, and he's great at letting me know that he loves and wants me."

Chapter 11

Designing Your Open Relationship

ONE OF THE MOST IMPORTANT requirements of an open relationship is that it be custom-tailored to the specific desires of the people involved. In this chapter, we'll explore what you need to bring your ideal open relationship to life, with exercises to help get you started as you draw the outline and fill in the details, then negotiate the design with your partner(s) and create rules, agreements, and a relationship contract.

Drawing the Outline

The style and structure of your relationship should reflect your personal values, philosophies, needs, desires, goals, and commitments. Before you think about all the specific details, decide first what the basic outline of your relationship looks like. Don't censor yourself: if you could have anything you wanted, what would it be? Do you want one committed partner with occasional sex mates? Multiple partners with whom you share sex, love, and romance? A network of sex buddies, but no serious relationship with anyone? A husband and a wife? Two husbands and a boyfriend? A BDSM play partner, a domestic partner, and a friend with benefits? Which of the styles in the previous chapters appeal to you, and why? Consider these statements and note the ones that resonate with you:

- I like the idea of sex with various people but having only one partner.
- I am committed to my partner, but I want to do BDSM with other people.
- I need to share an emotional connection with anyone I have a sexual relationship with.
- I can see myself committed/partnered/married to more than one person.
- I am open to the following elements in my relationships: sex, BDSM play, emotional connection, friendship, dating, romance, love, and commitment.
- I'm single and like to date a lot of people, but I don't want a serious partner.
- I would never want to live with a partner.
- Being in a relationship is not a high priority for me.
- If I found the right person, I could be in a committed relationship.
- I dislike the idea of hierarchy in relationships, with one partner primary and another secondary.
- I like each of my relationships to be clearly defined.
- I want to be someone's "number one" and vice versa.

Filling in the Details

Life is all about the details, and so is a successful open relationship. The following are some of the aspects you may want to think about as you design your open relationship, broken down into four categories: who (all about potential partners), what (activities and the nature of relationships), when (frequency and duration), and where (geography and logistics).

Some of these aspects may not matter to you at all, and that's okay. The details and the lists in the exercise that follow are meant to be exhaustive (though not definitive, of course). I have attempted to think of everything for you. It's impossible to negotiate with someone who says, "Anything is fine with me." You've got to get specific. Naturally, unforeseen issues will come up; perhaps it never occurred to you to ask your partner not to bring his other lovers to the local BDSM club, for example. But it happens, you get upset, you process it, and eventually amend the agreement. I would just like to save you time and get you thinking about these matters early on, in the hope of averting even one argument, one night of hurt and frustration, one misunderstanding.

You can't plan for everything: obstacles will still come up that you never talked about—that it never even occurred to you to discuss. Issues that you never anticipated will push your buttons. Behavior that you thought wouldn't make you jealous will. So, consider as many details as you can beforehand, and be ready for new ones to pop up.

Who: Gender, Characteristics, Roles, Familiarity

One of the first things to consider is who you (and your partners, if you have them) will be having sex with, dating, romancing, or forming a relationship with. Are there characteristics that limit your potential partners, such as gender, appearance, or age? For example, an agreement may be as straightforward as "no blondes" or "no one younger than me." Jimmy says all his relationships must "either serve my primary relationship or at least be neutral... I would probably be hesitant to engage with somebody who was a lot like [my primary]... I wouldn't duplicate her role." His primary partner is a dominant woman and a bondage expert. "If I were to take up with [another dominant female bondage expert], she'd kick my ass."

If you are bisexual or pansexual,[1] you and your partner may agree that you can have sex or relationships only with persons of the opposite gender. For example, Ginger and her husband have agreed that she can have as many female lovers as she wants but only one additional male lover. Bailey's partner is more comfortable with him playing with men than with other women.

An important issue to discuss is a potential partner's degree of familiarity. Can you have sex or form relationships with strangers, acquaintances, neighbors, co-workers, friends, ex-partners, a partner's relatives? For example, say you have a primary partner with sex mates on the side. You (or your partner) may prefer that you hook up with someone you don't know and your friends don't know; for some, this keeps their sex mates very separate from their lives. If this is a limit of yours, the sentiment is something like "I'd rather hook up with strangers or casual acquaintances"; if it reflects your partner's preference, it is more like "I don't want to know the people you have sex with." In the latter case, perhaps you would rather not encounter your partner's casual sex partners in your neighborhood, out at the local bar, or at the meeting of a group you belong to. If so, it's best to agree that your partner choose people outside your social circle. Depending on where you live, this may mean someone who is a stranger, belongs to a different community, or lives in a different town. Or maybe you don't mind if the person is a casual acquaintance or someone you see infrequently.

Having a relationship with a co-worker is tricky, since you usually have daily, extended contact with co-workers, making them impossible to avoid. Sleeping with or dating someone you work with can be complicated to begin with, and when you throw nonmonogamy into the mix, it can get even more dicey. First, some companies have explicit policies prohibiting office romances. As much as we might like to think that our personal relationships have no place at work, that's just not how it is. From company functions to water cooler chat, people tend to know who has a partner, who doesn't, and who's doing whom; if you bring your girlfriend to the annual holiday party and days later co-workers see you kissing the woman from accounting in the lobby, they will notice. The workplace can be a perfect environment for speculation, innuendo, and gossip. If you are not out about being in an open relationship, then people will assume you are cheating, which can affect people's perception of your character or ethics. If the

---

Who **Checklist**

(characteristics of potential partners)

Gender: ☐ women ☐ men ☐ transwomen/MTF
☐ transmen/FTM ☐ unimportant

Coupled status: ☐ single ☐ partnered ☐ unimportant

Sexual orientation: ☐ lesbian/gay/queer ☐ bisexual ☐
straight ☐ pansexual ☐ unimportant

S/M orientation: ☐ Top ☐ bottom ☐ switch ☐ unimportant

D/s orientation: ☐ Dominant ☐ submissive ☐ unimportant

Age: ☐ older ☐ younger ☐ approximately the same age
☐ unimportant

Familiarity: ☐ stranger ☐ unimportant

My: ☐ acquaintance ☐ best/close friend ☐ friend
☐ neighbor ☐ co-worker ☐ ex-partner

Partner's: ☐ acquaintance ☐ best/close friend ☐ friend
☐ neighbor ☐ co-worker ☐ ex-partner ☐ relative

Other characteristics:

  ☐ appearance:

  ☐ body type:

  ☐ identity (for example: swinger, crossdresser, butch)

dalliance or relationship ends, you must continue to work with the person, which can be stressful and painful—or awkward, at best. I am not saying that it can't be done. Plenty of folks have found nonmonogamous partners on the job and conducted casual or serious relationships with discretion and honor. But be forewarned that if you work with people you're involved with, it can get messy.

When it comes to friends as potential sex or relationship partners, everyone has a different philosophy. Some people are very clear on the division of friends and partners, as in: "These are my friends. I don't fuck my friends, and I don't want my partner(s) to fuck them either." If this statement rings true for you, it's important to make this clear to all your partners from the get-go. For people who value their friendships in this way and want to keep them entirely separate from romantic relationships, it can feel like a betrayal when a partner violates this boundary.

For others, it's the complete opposite: many of their friends *are* their lovers or partners. They tend to choose partners from within their social network or develop ongoing friendships with their sex mates, or both. Their partners know each other and may even have relationships with each other. They may be part of an extended yet tight-knit sub-community of people who have several partners in common, share each other's partners and ex-partners, and have close ties to one another. Chloe and her partner Dillon have a network of friends who are also lovers: "At this point, I have a request on the table that he not sleep with my girlfriend for my own psychological reasons: basically I feel like every single one of my female friends is banging him, so could I please have somebody in my life who is not banging him?" There is the potential for many thorny issues to come up whenever friendship is intertwined with a sexual relationship.

When it comes to choosing potential partners, ultimately, you and your partner(s) need to decide who is fair game and who is off limits. Often, our libido drives our choice, but I encourage you to step back from the situation if you can to make an honest evaluation of the person. There is no set of characteristics that describe the ideal secondary partner, boyfriend, play partner, sex buddy, or out-of-town fling; however, there are universal qualities you can look for.

You want someone who is self-aware, with strong communication skills, good boundaries, and a clear sense of who they are and what they want. If you have a primary relationship already, you want someone who will respect that relationship instead of attempting to break it up or otherwise wreak havoc on it. Trust your instincts and avoid people who will bring negative energy, a destructive agenda, unresolved baggage, or lots of drama to your life. Theo, a 46-year-old man, says about his current primary relationship of more than seven years: "There are people who are off limits: anyone who gives either of us an 'I don't like that person' vibe or anyone I can't trust to be in touch with their own feelings enough to handle a relationship like ours."

What: Sexual and BDSM Activities, Safer Sex, Romance

The content of a sexual encounter or relationship—what actually goes on between you and a partner—is one area where some nonmonogamous people may need or want to set limits for themselves and their partners. Think about what kinds of things you'd like to do with a new partner or partners and how you feel about what your partner does with other people. Are there limits when it comes to your sexual behavior with a potential partner, and if so, what are they? This covers a lot of terrain, from kissing to sex toys to dirty talk to anal sex. Perhaps you don't feel comfortable with your partner having vaginal intercourse with anyone but you, so that activity is off limits to others. Or you agree to play with others only when it involves your foot fetish, so there is no genital contact or sex at all. Here are some examples of people's limits.

What *Checklist*

(characteristics of potential interactions/relationships)

Interaction or relationship can include:

☐ affectionate and sexual activity (see checklist below for specifics)

☐ BDSM activity (specify)   ☐ socializing   ☐ friendship

☐ flirting   ☐ dating   ☐ courting/romance   ☐ sleepovers

☐ travel/vacation   ☐ emotional connection   ☐ love

☐ commitment   ☐ all of the above

☐ other:

Affectionate and Sexual Activities

Flirting   ☐ OK to give   ☐ OK to receive   ☐ not OK
☐ depends on:

Erotic touch (nongenital)   ☐ OK to give   ☐ OK to receive
☐ not OK   ☐ depends on:

Breast/nipple play   ☐ OK to give   ☐ OK to receive   ☐ not OK
☐ depends on:

Hand job/manual stimulation   ☐ OK to give   ☐ OK to receive
☐ not OK   ☐ depends on:

Frottage/tribadism   ☐ OK to give   ☐ OK to receive   ☐ not OK
☐ depends on:

Cunnilingus   ☐ OK to give   ☐ OK to receive   ☐ not OK
☐ depends on:

Fellatio   ☐ OK to give   ☐ OK to receive   ☐ not OK
☐ depends on:

Analingus   ☐ OK to give   ☐ OK to receive   ☐ not OK
☐ depends on:

Vaginal penetration with fingers   ☐ OK to give   ☐ OK to
receive   ☐ not OK   ☐ depends on:

Vaginal penetration with toys   ☐ OK to give   ☐ OK to receive
☐ not OK   ☐ depends on:

Vaginal penetration with penis □ OK to give □ OK to receive
□ not OK □ depends on:

Anal penetration with fingers □ OK to give □ OK to receive
□ not OK □ depends on:

Anal penetration with toys □ OK to give □ OK to receive
□ not OK □ depends on:

Anal penetration with penis □ OK to give □ OK to receive
□ not OK □ depends on:

Rough sex □ OK to give □ OK to receive □ not OK
□ depends on:

Spanking □ OK to give □ OK to receive □ not OK
□ depends on:

Bondage □ OK to give □ OK to receive □ not OK
□ depends on:

Erotic role play □ OK to give □ OK to receive □ not OK
□ depends on:

BDSM Activities
If you practice BDSM, make the same kind of list as above
with specific activities such as flogging, hot wax, Dominance
and submission.

As part of your discussion about sexual boundaries, you should
have a serious and specific talk about safer sex. To help guide you
through it, read Chapter 18, Safer Sex and Sexual Health.

*Individually, we can casually "fool around" with other people, that
is, we can do anything as long as there is no need for latex and we
stay in a public or otherwise peopled place (a bar or party—not
a private bedroom or other place where we would be alone with
the person).* —Sam

We can play with other people, but no vaginal or anal intercourse. There can be genital contact, orgasms, fisting, penetration with toys. —Sadie

If you have multiple relationships, you can also negotiate the nature of those relationships in terms of what I'll loosely call romantic/affectionate behavior. If you have a partner whom you see on a regular basis for sex, can you also go out on dates with him? What about sending naughty emails, flirting, courting, giving gifts, sleeping over, or traveling together? These are all things people who date do with one another, but you need to decide if they will be part of a relationship or not. For example, you may want to make the relationships other than your primary one solely about sex. Or, maybe you socialize as friends and hang out, but there are no love letters or flowers. It could be that you have sex and do some of the things listed, but consider what you have to be a friendship that's sexual. (Some call this "friends with benefits" or "sex buddies.")

We have no boundaries, we are each free to pursue whoever we want, whenever we want, and fall as deeply as the relationship takes us. We recognize where we are in our life, how close we feel, how much time is available, so we don't enter into relationships when they might negatively impact our primary relationship.
—Ilana and Luke

Who and What for BDSM Players

Those BDSM practitioners who emphasize the D/s of BDSM thrive on relationship power dynamics. Because the roles they take on are clearly (or some would say rigidly) defined, it gives each person a specific set of expectations. But it also limits the relationship to that particular dynamic. If you want to explore another part of your identity or a different dynamic, you can do so with other people. For example, you are the submissive in your relationship with your Dominant, D. You'd like to try your hand at topping someone, but that is not part of your dynamic with D. So, you open your relationship to include play and even other relationships to explore a chance for you to be the top. I can be a Master and have a slave and a girl, the girl can have a Daddy, and my slave could herself be Mistress to a girl. Who everyone is to one another is clear and very distinct.

As an extension of this style, you can create some form of role exclusivity within your nonmonogamy. Role exclusivity can help people feel that they know exactly where they stand and potentially mitigate some kinds of jealousy. For example, as a Dominant, Jimmy has a boy, Jay. Jimmy may play with other submissives and even other boys, but no one else is *his* boy. This in turn gives Jay a sense of security about his specific, special place in Jimmy's life. As Jimmy says:

I've found that by defining the relationships in some way distinct from other relationships, there's a greater sense of safety and comfort. Jay as my boy is the boy, the only boy. There are times when other people serve me, there are times when other people do any of the things that he does for me, but they aren't mine. I am committed to not having another boy, and he's committed to not having another sir.

My primary and I had a kinky relationship, a Daddy/girl bond. We agreed that while other men could top me, no one else could be my Daddy. —Barbara

Similarly, some people who switch between top and bottom negotiate that when they play with others they can assume a role different from their usual role with their primary partner. For instance, let's say you have a BDSM relationship with your partner. You are the Top and she is the bottom. You've agreed that when you play with others, you can bottom to them. Your partner is comfortable when you play with others because it doesn't call into question her role as "your bottom"; she doesn't feel she is competing with your other partners because they're not bottoms when they play with you.

When: Frequency, Specific Days or Times

If you've agreed that you and your partner can have one-time hookups, then the issue of ongoing contact with an additional partner is moot. But if you have ongoing relationships with other people, you need to decide on the guidelines for how much regular contact you or your partner have with others. This gets to the core of one of the essential elements in negotiating nonmonogamy: managing your time. Your heart may have endless love to give and you may have copious amounts of energy to put into relationships, but there are only 24 hours in a day. How much of that 24 hours you spend with a partner—whether online, by phone, or in person—is an important consideration. Would you prefer if your partner had infrequent contact with her sex buddies and only talked to them to set up dates? Will you talk to a partner every day?

In addition, how much time will you spend with a partner? Will you see someone once a week, once a month, every three months? Do you want to set a minimum and maximum amount of time you spend with a partner you don't live with? Think about what you are comfortable with. Can you go out with another partner, but no more than twice a week? Are there specific limits you want to set for when you can have sex or a date with a partner? For example, maybe you can have hookups only when you and your primary partner are geographically separated, when one of you is out of town, say. You might decide that Friday nights are reserved for you and your primary partner. Perhaps you share custody of children with an ex-spouse and negotiate that if you or your current partner wants to sleep over elsewhere, it can only be when the kids are not with you.

Where: Geography, Events, Home

Are there limits about where you have sex or dates with a potential partner? Many people choose to design their nonmonogamy around geography to define it as separate from the primary relationship. For example, one partner may say, "You can have a girlfriend as long as she lives in another town." Or: "Each of us travels a lot for business, and when we're away from home, we can have flings." If you live in a small town, often you must be extremely discreet about your open relationships. If this is the case, you may agree that other partners, whether one-time or recurring, must live elsewhere and dates must take place somewhere other than your hometown. Ilana says, "We have had concerns about getting involved with someone locally, in part because this is a small town and we aren't out in the community, and in part because of anticipated time and energy concerns."

For some people, exploring sex with others is specific to a place. You can play with other people only when you go to clubs, parties, or events; this is especially true for swingers and BDSMers. It is often these environments that are conducive to such exploration, since they are sexually charged, the majority of the attendees are part of a community, and many people are there specifically to find other partners.

If several of your partners live in the same area, you have other issues to ponder. If you live with one partner, can you have another partner over to the house for a date, or is that off limits? How do you feel about either of you having sex with another partner in the bed you share? Many people reported having a separate bedroom or playroom for other partners or activities because they agreed their bedroom was off limits.

Sex in our bed is okay, but sex in the meditation room is completely off limits. My room is mine. He is not allowed to have sex in there. Likewise with me in his room. —Elizabeth

Negotiation

Negotiation is one of the most important steps in designing your open relationship. I simply do not believe in attitudes such as "Let's just see how it goes," "We can decide on a case-by-case basis," or "We'll make it up as we go along." I am all for spontaneity, but not when it comes to people's relationship values and boundaries. You want to go into an open relationship with very clear intentions and limits. You want to have those intentions and limits articulated, and in doing so, leave nothing unsaid. Nothing should be *implied* in the negotiation process; it should all be spelled out. Neglecting to anticipate and make decisions about important issues in advance can be a recipe for disaster.

Begin your negotiation process from a place of stability. If you have unresolved issues with a partner or are in a state of transition, it's not a good time to create a radical structure change or commit to another partner. Aiden, an FTM living with two women, always checks in with other members of the triad before dating someone new. "We talk with each other and make sure everyone's in a good place. We've learned not to bring a new person into the mix when one person is already feeling insecure or their needs aren't getting met." George, a computer engineer from Minneapolis, agrees that timing is important, and he likes to err on the side of caution when adding a new partner. "If the underlying individual relationships can't support the weight, the whole thing will crack."

The best time to negotiate is when you are clear-headed and feeling good about the relationship. It's a bad idea to negotiate and make decisions when you are fighting or don't feel secure about yourself or the relationship. It's also difficult, though not impossible, to negotiate when you've developed a crush on a new person or someone is waiting in the wings for you to open up your relationship. If you are going to an event where you hope to hook up—a private party, a sex or swing club, a conference, a resort—always negotiate before you get there.

When *Checklist*

Frequency of contact:
☐ one time only

☐ ongoing, infrequent, specify:

☐ ongoing, frequent, specify:

☐ other:

☐ all of the above

☐ Are there special occasions or days of the week reserved for a particular partner? (specify)

Where *Checklist*

☐ out of town

☐ in town

☐ public settings (parties, clubs)

☐ events

☐ at home

☐ not at home

☐ other:

There is nothing worse than finding someone you are interested in, then having to stop flirting, pull your partner to the side, and say, "So what is okay here and what's not?" It breaks the flow, it's inappropriate, and you're already caught up in a sexually charged atmosphere. With your judgment affected by lust, you may not make the best decision.

Approach the negotiation process with an open heart and mind and with honesty and trust. Trust that your partner has good intentions. This is not about one-upping each other or winning the negotiation. Each of you should feel that you have been respected and treated fairly, that the rules set forth are fair. No one has been set up to fail. Each of you is getting most of what you want and need, and you are able to compromise in certain areas where necessary. No one feels pressured or coerced to agree to something. Each of you has a voice in the process.

When a new issue comes up, give yourself time to decide. If a partner comes to you to check in about a new partner, don't feel compelled to say yes or no right away. My partner and I have agreed to check in with each other before we hook up with someone else, and I've been guilty of jumping to yes before I've given a situation enough thought. My intentions are good: I say yes because I want to support my partner's sexual adventures. But now, instead of jumping to yes, I say, Give me a day (or an hour or a week) to think about it. Taking time makes us both feel better: I get a chance to ponder the situation, and my partner feels confident in my decision because he knows it's a thoughtful one.

I discuss below some things to consider during your negotiation, such as veto power, prior permission, separate versus together, and interaction between partners. Many of these points are very practical, but don't mistake practical for insignificant. Any of these issues can carry an emotional wallop. You must be sensitive, and remember that an issue that matters little to you could mean a great deal to someone else.

Prior Permission or Notification

Do you need prior permission from a primary (or other) partner before you pursue someone else? Do you need someone's okay for certain sexual activities, but not others? Perhaps casual experiences can be allowed to happen spontaneously, but you need to inform a partner or partners about the potential for an ongoing relationship. Some people want to be informed about any new partner beforehand, like Ilana and Luke: "We always attempt to discuss it with each other before entering into a new relationship, to give our partner an opportunity to ask questions, raise concerns, and to get comfortable with whatever level of risk a partner may be." Some prefer to know in advance but allow for spontaneous opportunities. Elizabeth says, "We try to give each other a heads-up before we do anything, but we recognize that it may not be possible in the moment, so we trust each other to make the right decision." Many people say that while they don't give or get permission, they appreciate being kept in the loop so they feel informed about what's going on in their partners' lives.

Veto Power over New Partners

Veto power is the ability to say no to a potential new partner and have it respected, no matter what. Some believe that veto power is an essential component to making nonmonogamous relationships work. While certain couples want to have a discussion about the veto, others say they trust each other to use the veto wisely, no questions asked. Some partners who have veto power built into their agreement say that it has rarely been used, but when it has, it has been honored. For those who believe strongly in it, veto power provides reassurance that each partner has a voice at this important moment. Dahlia says: "My spouse and I always talk if we are interested in playing with a prospective partner. We describe the new person, share our thoughts, concerns, and desires. If either of us says no about a potential fuck buddy, then we are to respect that decision. We want to make sure that our extracurricular activities are loads of fun, but do not compromise our primary relationship."

Some of the folks I interviewed said that while they don't believe in veto power, if a partner raised a concern, they would listen to their issues and seriously consider their feelings. They don't see this as a veto, because they don't believe a partner should have such absolute, no-questions-asked power. Eli says: "I prefer to think of this as 'preferring each other's approval' as opposed to either of us exercising a veto."

Others reject the notion of veto altogether and consider it a problematic concept. These folks don't believe in putting limits on their partners. They don't feel it is their prerogative to stop their partner from pursuing an experience or relationship, and they want the same freedom in return. Barbara is a bisexual woman from Columbus, Ohio:

> *This is one area that caused my primary and me the most pain in our relationship. I understood that there was veto power, that if a relationship caused one of us enough pain, the other would end it. It was even proof in some way that we were primary to each other. But when I used it to veto someone, the real-life run caused a lot of pain. I broke my own rule of everyone taking care of their own needs. By using the veto, I made him responsible for my needs; he refused to, and it crushed me. I would never accept or negotiate veto power again in any relationship. I would listen and consider my partner's side, and expect a good deal of listening and processing, but in the end everyone makes their own choices.*

Chloe, 29, and Dillon, 39, are relationship coaches who have been together for four years and live in New York City. Chloe is adamantly against veto power: "I think the concept of veto power in some ways encourages people to just hold on to things until they are so agitated that they want to veto." Her partner Dillon agrees: "For some people the only way to make things safe is to actually throw up a wall. The more savvy you are in taking care of your own needs and the more savvy you are at making yourself feel safe, the less you need veto power."

Ultimately, I think, veto power can be a useful tool if it's used correctly. Be clear about what it means and why you want it: you are asking for and giving your partner the authority to nix a partner. It does make some people feel safe and reassures them that their relationship is a priority, and it can be helpful if you are just trying out nonmonogamy. Veto power should not be put in place so that you can avoid processing your underlying feelings or dealing with jealousy. It should not be used arbitrarily or abused just because you don't like someone in a superficial way.

The notion of veto power raises a broader issue: what happens when you don't agree with your partner's choice of other partners? It would be wonderful if we met all our partner's partners and totally loved them, but that is not always the case. Sometimes you meet a person your partner totally digs, and you just can't see the appeal. Maybe the new person rubs you the wrong way, raises a red flag, or sets off an alarm. Whatever you want to call it, you just don't like him. If you know the person disrespects you or your relationship, then it's absolutely valid to raise this as a serious concern. If you think the person lies about safer sex practices and is going to put you at risk, bring it up. But if you just think the person is immature, annoying, or a drama queen, it's much trickier.

We don't want to see our partners get hurt. We want to give them good advice. We don't want to have to pick up the pieces of an explosion we could have predicted from day one. The truth is that sometimes we have to sit by and let the ones we love make mistakes and get involved in bad relationships. Be loving, be supportive, and keep an open mind. If the shit hits the fan, no I-told-you-so's.

Separate or Together

For some nonmonogamous partners, the presence or involvement of each partner in romantic or sexual encounters is another issue to think about. When you have sex or a date with another person, would you like your primary partner to be there? Some folks, like a couple I met in Boston years ago, adopt a simple rule: "We are a package deal." They had sex with others together as a couple; neither partner ever went off on their own. If you are turned on by watching your partner have sex with another person or being watched as you do the same, sticking together is a good option for you. Some people say that being present and involved helps alleviate their fear and insecurity: if you're not there, your mind can run wild with what might be happening. Another couple was at the other end of the spectrum: "If she wants to hook up with someone else, I generally would rather not be around. We once hooked up with another couple—she went with the husband and I went with the wife. Just hearing her in the next room with him made me really jealous; that's when I realized I didn't want to be there."

August and Stacy have been in a polyamorous relationship for five years. On this particular issue, the two are very different. Stacy says, "August is better with the in-your-face poly. He has no issues seeing me cuddle or have sex with my partners, but I am very uncomfortable seeing him with his lovers. I guess what I mean is that August has very few jealousy triggers and I have quite a few. Working around them has been difficult, and I often feel hypocritical asking him not to do something when he would have no issue with me doing it." August gives some background: "Stacy and I figured out the 'no sex in front of Stacy' rule largely by accident, a couple years ago. After holding a sex party at my house one weekend, she took off and then came back later to find me in bed with someone else. We weren't doing anything, but it freaked her out and there was massive drama and crying. This was despite the fact that she had watched me have sex with others at the party earlier in the weekend—once the context was outside of the party, things were different. Since then we've stuck to a 'no sex in front of Stacy' rule in most cases, which has prevented a reoccurrence."

All three of us enjoy watching each other with other partners, so we like to be there for it. Sometimes we will join in, other times the two of us not participating will just watch and snuggle. All of us must be present when sex occurs outside the triad. —Owen

Site-specific Play

If you and your partner like to attend sex or BDSM parties, clubs, or events, then you may want to begin your exploration of non-monogamy by making it "site-specific." Think of this as nonmonogamy's version of the popular tourism slogan "What happens in Vegas stays in Vegas." You can agree to explore experiences with other people only in a particular location (whatever your version of Vegas is). Usually, these spaces are very erotically charged and provide an opportunity—for the evening or a weekend—to step outside your everyday lives as exclusive partners.

Such an open environment can help to ignite your sex drive and lower your inhibitions, but remember that this doesn't mean anything goes. You must negotiate limits and make an agreement beforehand and stick to it. You should decide if you want to meet people and accompany them to a hotel or somewhere else private, or you prefer to play in a public space where others can watch.

While the idea of being watched may scare the crap out of you, for some people what happens in public feels safer than what happens in private, for a variety of reasons. First, you can watch or be nearby when your partner is with someone else, which for some people is a big turn-on; this also means you don't have to worry about your partner's physical safety. At an established event, you're more likely to encounter people experienced in nonmonogamy and you have the opportunity to hook up with people you don't have any social ties to. And some people feel the public aspect is lighter, more sociable, and less threatening than a one-on-one encounter in private.

When extracurricular experiences happen at specific places, they feel more contained: we went, we met some people, we played, we came home together. This is not just for beginners: plenty of nonmonogamy veterans stick to this site-specific model, since it keeps the focus on the primary relationship while allowing for additional experiences on special occasions under special circumstances.

Sharing Information

After a one-time experience or as part of an ongoing affair, will you kiss and tell? And how much information will you share about other experiences and partners? This is an especially important point to discuss if you have a primary partner. You need to determine your comfort level with sharing intimate details—both as the one who shares them and the one who hears them. Think carefully about whether you'll share these details, what you will tell each other and what you won't, what you'd like to know and what you wouldn't.

Some partners may want to know only the basics: I had sex with this woman in Philadelphia. The more details you supply, the more there is to fret, worry, or get jealous over; so the less they know, the better. Or, they may simply not be interested.

Others want more detail because they want to be kept in the loop, but they also want to respect each other's privacy to some extent. Shari says she and her husband are open with each other about other partners:

While the "in love" feelings are reserved for each other, we are not threatened by other feelings of closeness, or intense bonding, connected to other partners. We are aroused by seeing the other happy and turned on to a person and like to hear about each other's solo dates, but only to a point. We allow each other to have emotional privacy and understand that the other partners touch us in ways we can't with each other. We're happy that we each have others in our lives who can do this for and with us.

Some people want *all* the details. This can fulfill two very different desires: putting a partner's mind at ease and turning them on. For some, knowing the specifics helps mitigate their fear and jealousy:

I want to know the details about any emotional interest, entanglements, infatuations that she is feeling. And I will listen to as much detail about her sexual attraction toward someone as that other partner is comfortable with me knowing about. I try very, very hard, sometimes not very successfully, to be respectful of other peoples' boundary stuff about that. I have a general nosiness thing going on. The more I know, the less I worry… I can tell the

*degree of how invested in the relationship she is and how much
I need to get to know that person. I don't usually have lots of
problems with jealousy and insecurity but when they do come up
it's when I don't know a lot about what's going on. If I feel really
left out of the loop about what's going on, then I will invent something, which is scary and threatening at that point. And if I know,
then almost always it's fine and nice and good.* —Pat

For others, sharing details—specifically of sexual encounters—is
a turn-on. Ophelia says, "When it comes to my sexual adventures, I
always tell him the really juicy details while we are having sex; we both
enjoy that."

If you are not sure how much to tell a partner, ask him and get a
clear answer. And keep in mind that what you want to know and what
he wants to know can change. Check in often to get a sense of how
your information sharing is working for both of you.

Interaction Between Partners

What kind of relationship, if any, will there be among your different
partners? Do you want them to meet each other once, but that's all? Are
they part of the same community, so seeing each other frequently is
inevitable? Is it important to you that they get along? Do you want
them to be friends? Are you okay if they become lovers? People have
lots of opinions on this subject.

*There's a need-to-know level. But there's definitely not a need-to-
like level. I don't have to fuck them.* —Kathleen

*We may not really like each other but we respect each other's
place in his life.* —Lena

*My partners meeting and getting to know one another is very
important to me.* —Marcus

If it's somebody that [my primary partner] has a really serious relationship with, then I think it's absolutely required—in order for things to function well—for me to have a good relationship with that person too. —Pat

Shari, 48, is an adult entertainer, educator, and author whose marriage is nonmonogamous. She makes an important point about privacy and discretion and how it can help facilitate partners getting along with each other: "Our other partners know of each other, certainly. Our female partners do know each other from work [in the adult industry]. We never talk about one playmate to another, or what we do, or how we feel about her, to any of the others. We keep each one pretty private. This is an important aspect of why it works. Each relationship is its own thing, and each woman is her own person, with her own charms, needs, and compatibilities. We treat them like the individuals they are. This way, we can all be in the same room and there's no unpleasant energy flying around."

Rules and Agreements

Our primary rule is not "anything goes," it's "everything is negotiable." —Owen

Everyone is responsible for getting their own needs met. —Barbara

I will generally not make agreements in relationships that do not permit me to express myself in a way that feels authentic to me. If I do, then I am prone to resentment if it continues. —Kathleen

Rules outline behavior, reflect each person's limits and boundaries, and spell out the expectations that all parties have agreed to. Rules help guide people to know what's okay and what's not. Rules allow people to feel safe, reassured, and secure, and thus they are an important tool in creating successful open relationships. Many people are comfortable with the term *rules* and its associated meanings, while others don't like the word itself. They believe that rules are about confining, controlling, and limiting people's behavior, and they don't wish to do this to their partners. Whether you embrace the concept of rules or not, it's important to come up with a set of terms and guidelines, agree to them, and honor your agreement. What you agree on could be typed on six single-spaced pages, hashed over in a series of emails, or boiled down to one or two verbal statements you make to one another.

Keep in mind that some of your guidelines may determine or inform others. For example: if you hook up with someone while you're out of town, I don't need to meet her; but if you're going to have an ongoing sex buddy in town, I want to be introduced. Along these lines, existing rules and boundaries that you have with one partner may limit or even define the rules you have with another.

Here are some examples of people's rules and agreements:

We practice safer sex religiously and get comprehensive testing on a regular basis. We let each other know if we'll be out, out later than expected, or out all night. —Pat

No other relationship is allowed to harm ours. We tell each other about new people before anything happens below the belt. —Cheryl

If we go to a play/sex party together, we play together. —Stacy

No drama; no love affairs; no lying or withholding important information; no crazy people. There is no sexual limit to behavior; if it's hot for all involved, we support going for it. —Shari

If someone asks for reassurance, it is in your best interests to give it. A lot of drama and hurt feelings can be avoided if this step is honored. Recognizing that insecurity will happen, taking the time to reassure someone of their place in your life can go a long way toward acceptance. —Bella

Agreements are about respecting boundaries; they are not about control. Agreements are not about avoiding the difficult stuff. Don't agree to something because you think it will protect your partner from feeling jealous or having to deal with her own issues. Agreements are ultimately about making people feel safe, secure, and reassured.

While I recommend laying out specific guidelines, I want to acknowledge that there those who do not subscribe to this practice and believe strongly that rules are not useful to or conducive to an open relationship.

The Myth of Equality

The women's movement has had a tremendous impact on the way people behave in relationships, especially with respect to gender. For too long, it was assumed and expected that people would take on certain responsibilities—breadwinner, homemaker, parent, caretaker—based on rigidly defined roles of "husband" and "wife." Early feminist thought challenged that notion and argued that we should strive for more equal partnerships. The idea of equality has subtly seeped into our collective consciousness and produced some important shifts in expectations and opportunities for people of all genders. But it has also become part of the unspoken script for the modern relationship. People assume everyone should have equality in their relationships; if they don't, someone is getting the short end of the stick. Every partner in a relationship absolutely should have an equal right to consent, negotiate, and be heard. But some people have confused equality with symmetry, making the assumption that everyone should have the same thing.

Morgan, a male crossdresser from New York City, says, "In my opinion the hardest thing is establishing a sense of symmetry or reciprocity in the nonmonogamy. By that I mean: it's going to work best if *both* partners are playing with others, rather than just one of them while the other tolerates the situation. So perhaps the only potential tension in my relationship with Dahlia is the fact that I occasionally meet with people on my own and she (almost) never has."

When it comes to designing your open relationship, don't let the ideal of equality trip you up. As you negotiate the details of a relationship, you must acknowledge that you and a partner are two people with different personal styles and needs, some—but not all—of which may overlap. Sometimes, setting the same rules for both partners simply doesn't make sense, because you are different people who want different things. For instance, having a rule that you can only sleep with men outside the relationship wouldn't work if one partner is a bisexual woman and the other is a straight man. You may be a person who enjoys safe, anonymous sex, or one who can't imagine it. You may like to take time to get to know a potential sexual partner, or you may get off on public sex. Perhaps you want a relationship before you become intimate, or you are looking for a long-term Dominant/submissive dynamic. In one couple I know, the wife loves to go to swingers' clubs, orgies, and sex parties and have public sex, whereas the husband likes to have girlfriends to romance: women he can take on dates, travel with, and fawn over. Different needs require different guidelines for each person. Pat, a women's health clinic coordinator from Ohio, talks about how she and her girlfriend differ:

> I tend more toward suddenly falling into relationships or having infrequent but ongoing sexual contacts with good friends. Ellen tends toward more casual, "just met you but you seem nice" sex. There would be no way to keep those kinds of things even, it would just be silly. Ellen is much more interested in sexual relationships with people with whom she does not have an ongoing relationship of some kind than I could possibly imagine myself being.

Each partner deserves equal respect, of course, but equality, in the sense of who gets to do what with whom, can be unreasonable and unrealistic for some people. How many couples do you know where both partners contribute the same amount of time, money, housecleaning, gardening skill, cooking, parenting, travel planning, emotional energy, romance, and erotic inspiration? If you extend this to the terms of your open relationship, a rule such as "If I have two girlfriends, then you should have two girlfriends" may sound like an attractive idea, but in reality life seldom works that way. In attempting to give each partner an equal amount of freedom, you could lose sight of what each person actually wants. Instead, see what you can do to accommodate people's different personal styles and desires.

Work to achieve balance, rather than equality. This is not simply a matter of semantics; there is a difference. Balance means that everyone is generally getting their needs met; no one is compromising too much or feeling too limited by the agreement. All partners have agreed to priorities concerning the time and energy they dedicate to the relationship, and each partner's actions reflect these priorities. No one feels taken advantage of.

The Relationship Contract

As part of the negotiation process for a BDSM scene or a relationship, some kinky people write and sign a contract to outline their limits and what they've agreed to. Even if you are uninterested in BDSM, I recommend you borrow this practice from the world of BDSM. A relationship contract can be a useful tool in negotiating your nonmonogamy. This contract is not a legal document, but rather a written agreement in which you clearly articulate your needs, wants, limits, rules, expectations, goals, and commitments.

Writing a contract is a helpful exercise for really nailing down what you want; it may get you thinking about things you never considered. One of the benefits of a contract is that it makes the terms of your relationship real; it can strengthen your bond, since you commit to what you put on paper and to each other. It can help prevent miscommunication, and it can serve as a reference point for resolving it, especially when people don't remember exactly what was said about a particular issue ("I thought you said—" "I thought you meant—"). Trust me, it's much better to ask for clarification when you're negotiating the contract rather than when you're in a hotel room about to have sex with someone! You can return to the contract periodically to check in with each other and revise your agreement.

Here are some elements you can incorporate into a relationship contract:

- A statement about the nature of your relationship and your commitment to one another
- A statement about your personal values and philosophies
- What you hope to achieve through nonmonogamy
- The rules or guidelines for: who, what, when, where, other partners, safe sex
- Other pertinent limits and boundaries
- Schedule of time and date commitments
- The process for starting a relationship with a new partner
- The process for airing grievances
- Agreement about being "out" to other people
- Explanation of how to amend the agreement

While a contract can clarify your agreement and commitment to one another, it is not a guarantee of anything. A contract will not make your nonmonogamous relationship perfect. A contract cannot prevent miscommunication, misunderstanding, or irresponsible or hurtful behavior. It should not be used to justify behavior after the fact: "Our contract didn't say anything about strippers in other countries." The contract is a tool for communication and clarification, not a weapon to be wielded against someone later. No matter how thorough you are, a situation will probably arise that is not covered by the contract; remember that it's not only about what is on paper in black and white, it's about the *spirit* of the contract. While a contract can bring clarity, it is not meant to set anything in stone. Your relationship, limits, and boundaries will change—your desires and sexuality may change subtly or dramatically—and your agreements should change with them. For more on coping with changes and renegotiating your agreements, see Chapter 15, Opening Up Again: When Something Changes.

PROFILE: IGNACIO AND KHANE

> *"We made a conscious decision to be primaries—*
> *to create a spiritual base."*

IGNACIO AND KHANE, BOTH 35, live in Brooklyn with Ignacio's daughter, whom they are raising together. Ignacio, who is African American and Puerto Rican, works as a sex worker, educator, and performance artist. Khane, who is African American, is a store manager and entrepreneur. They are queer. "We were identified female at birth," Khane says. "We say we are trans-entities. We are both male and female, and neither. We both use male pronouns because we are not fond of the gender-neutral ones, *ze/hir,*[2] and using solely female pronouns is not what we desire. We navigate through the world in which some people see us as guys, others as gals, and others don't know."

Their relationship began five years ago as friends and fuck buddies. After three years together, things began to shift, but neither of them wanted a primary partner because of their past experiences. They say they resisted calling each other primaries even as friends and family saw them as such. Ignacio says: "We finally said, let's just call it what it is and let's dive headfirst into [it] and see what happens. I don't want to pretend that this isn't happening. I want to be conscious about it. Let's name it and do it, and if it doesn't work, it doesn't work."

They began negotiating their respective boundaries. Khane says, "We started out with quite a few rules and boundaries that helped us to gain trust and figure out how we could maintain our polyamorous relationship in an open and healthy way. We started with boundaries around seeing people in the workplace. We placed expectations about respect from other lovers. We had boundaries around not sleeping [over with other partners]. There were many that came and faded away just as fast as they were made... I think we started out with a lot because of our fears. Because we jumped into being primaries, we [wanted to] be completely cautious about things."

Ignacio explains what being primaries means to them today: "My relationship with Khane is primary because we made a conscious decision to be primaries—to create a spiritual base. We run a household together, pay bills together, but we don't consider that the base of our primary status. It is based in spirituality, vulnerability, [a] high level of intimacy, friendship, and struggle." Khane adds: "We have put a lot of work into our relationship through constant communication, and because of that we are able to open up to others. I love having my foundation. I love that I have found someone who can be my friend, lover, partner, fuck buddy, BDSM partner at any given time and still be polyamorous."

They do not have veto power over potential partners. However, because they practice BDSM together, they agreed that when they are in play spaces, if someone wants to top Ignacio, Khane must give them permission. When Ignacio is on his own, he can choose to be dominated, with the caveat that he tell the person that his Master is Khane. "We negotiate constantly and always leave everything open for discussion. We both like knowing we are not stuck in one way of being. Some boundaries are made just until we get over a phobia we may have developed from a past relationship that went bad. That's how we heal each other," Khane says.

As a couple, they have a relationship with Chandra. Ignacio says, "I was co-workers with her for a couple of months and got to know her as a friend. She attended one of my play parties and got into a really sexy scene with Khane. I was so turned on by it that I initiated a three-way date. Since then, we have grown in a relationship with her. It has been challenging at times but we are always so amazed at how we are able to function, check ourselves, and grow together as a three-way and separately."

When Khane feels jealous, he says, "I allow myself to feel it. Then I figure out where it's coming from and why. Sometimes I tell Ignacio about it and sometimes I just process myself through it and let it go. Most times it has to do with the frustration of not having a date with Ignacio in a while or needing him to fuck me, or needing to dominate him. In the end, it is usually not attached to the other person at all. On those rare occasions where it is pure jealousy, we process it and figure if it's a matter of renegotiating something, strengthening some part of our foundation, or just realizing it's something that will only go away with time, like getting used to a new situation."

When Ignacio and Khane first became primaries, they decided to create something called Alone Month, an entire month dedicated to the relationship, during which they would not see any other partners. Ignacio explains: "We picked August because our anniversary is in August. We decided that we have to find a time in the year when we come together and just concentrate on our foundation. If we don't do that, it'll fall apart—that's the only way we'll maintain being together. So we do a lot of spiritual work. We do a body cleansing, internal work, baths, going to the ocean, feeding the gods, and working on our altar. We develop our role-play characters and just concentrate on having lots and lots of sex, lots and lots of conversations, and renegotiating."

Chapter 12

Jealousy and Other Intense Feelings

PEOPLE HAVE LOTS of different theories about love and relationship dynamics. I am not going to go into healing your inner child, reenacting parent/child dynamics, getting the love you want, or how to love without losing yourself—all that terrain and more has been covered elsewhere. I believe the bottom line is this: relationships raise issues. Relationships give us the chance to experience deep connection and intimacy, intense bonding, understanding, and unconditional love. They can be supportive, exhilarating, healing, and magical. At the same time, relationships are like cauldrons: ideal places to throw two (or more) people's issues together, and see what mixes, bubbles up, or explodes.

In relationships, we get our buttons pushed, emotional baggage revealed, inner demons confronted, and old wounds ripped open—we experience every emotion in the book. Relationships can be difficult, overwhelming, frustrating, and painful. Ultimately, they give us the chance to change old patterns, to become stronger, to learn and grow. It's this opportunity for personal growth that makes relationships worth the hard work we put into them. And make no mistake: relationships take lots of work. When you have an open relationship—whether it's partnered nonmonogamy, polyamory, or some other style—the issues increase exponentially. Add more people to the mix, and along with them come their problems, fears, hot buttons, and baggage.

The first step to learning and growing is self-awareness and the willingness to tackle your own issues and limitations. I will go so far as to say that self-awareness is a prerequisite for positive relationships— and most definitely for positive nonmonogamous relationships. Relationships demand that you learn to become aware of your feelings and communicate them, which means being vulnerable and sharing your darkest fears and insecurities. The best way to conquer your fears is to shine a light on them and talk about them. It's a challenge, but a rewarding one. The more clear you become about who you are, what you want, and what makes you tick emotionally, the better a relation-ship partner you will be. The work begins with yourself. I won't prescribe how you work on yourself—you may choose counseling, support groups, a self-help program, meditation, journaling, spiritual work, a combination of these, or something else entirely—but I recom-mend that you do.

People who practice nonmonogamy face all kinds of issues in their relationships. However, as a general rule, some common feelings arise, including jealousy, fear of abandonment, and resentment. I'll explore the origins and complexities of these feelings and suggest ways to deal with them.

Jealousy

One of the questions people in open relationships are asked most often is "Don't you get jealous?" We experience jealousy in all kinds of situ-ations, and it is especially charged in love and sexual relationships. Some people believe that jealousy is "natural," but I think of it more as a learned, nearly universal behavior. It is a key emotion that almost everyone has felt at some point. Jealousy drives the plots of ancient myth, classical and modern literature, drama, and opera. It is also one of the integral assumptions of monogamy: society teaches us that we're *supposed* to be jealous when a partner flirts with someone else, another suitor pursues him, or he falls in love with another person. In their book *The Myth of Monogamy*, David P. Barash and Judith Eve Lipton report that "the most common cause of one spouse killing another is sexual jealousy, specifically a man's suspicion that his mate has been unfaithful."[1]

Among the people I interviewed, there are two schools of thought about feeling jealous. Some say that they rarely, if ever, experience the emotion. Take, for example, Morgan, a 48-year-old professor who identifies as a bisexual crossdresser, and his wife, Dahlia, a 40-year-old bisexual professor. They have been together for eight years and have an open relationship style that resembles partnered nonmonogamy. "Once Dahlia and I became secure about each other's commitment to the relationship, any feelings of jealousy vanished. At least they did for me," Morgan says. Dahlia concurs. "[Jealous feelings] are wasted emotions and a complete waste of my time. I trust my spouse completely, so I really don't experience these feelings. My spouse has never given me reason to feel these emotions, well, at least not in relation to our lifestyle... With others, if they show signs of jealousy or possessiveness, the relationship gets severed immediately. Usually, though, our fuck buddies know the rules and don't engage in such emotions."

> "Why should sex of all things be the thing that breaks up relationships and causes such jealousy when a good conversation can go deeper, TV can steal more of your attention, and chess (as I found toward the end of one relationship) can take your lover away from you for longer."
>
> —ALISON ROWAN[2]

On the other side of the coin are interviewees who acknowledge that jealousy is an issue they struggle with. Some believe it is a learned behavior that can be unlearned, and they work hard to rise above jealousy and eradicate it from their lives. Others work to discover why they get jealous and deal with the source of the jealousy. For experienced nonmonogamists, jealousy usually rears its head at predictable moments: when a new person enters the picture, when a casual partner becomes more serious, or when some significant change happens.

I don't tend to be jealous as long as I feel as though I am getting "enough" attention, energy, time. If I feel jealous for more than a little flash, that's a sign that I feel like I'm getting less than I want or expect, which means it's time to have a chat. —Duke

Many people, even poly people, seem terrified of jealousy... I think of jealousy as the warning light on your dashboard. It tells you something is wrong, but doesn't tell you what to do about it. When you feel jealousy, it means it's time to pull over and assess what is going on, and only then do something about it. —Owen

Jealousy is really an umbrella term for a constellation of feelings including envy, competitiveness, insecurity, inadequacy, possessiveness, fear of abandonment, feeling unloved, and feeling left out. To say simply "I am jealous" is far too vague, since it means different things to different people and it manifests itself in so many diverse ways. Like Owen's "warning light," it's more useful to think of jealousy as a sign that something's not right. Try to figure out exactly what you're feeling, the root(s) of the feeling, and what you need to feel better. Digging around can open a Pandora's box, but until you realize why you're jealous you will not be able to resolve the issues causing the feeling. Once you identify the source of the jealousy, you will be better able to cope with it, feel less controlled and motivated by it, and you may be able to let go of it altogether. Below I discuss four specific emotions as the components of jealousy: envy, insecurity, possessiveness, and feeling excluded.

Envy

When you experience envy, you want something that someone else has: it could be a physical object, but in relationships it's more likely to be a personality trait, another relationship, or a certain dynamic between two people. The grass is greener on the other side of the fence: you feel that you are not as good as someone else, what you have is not as good as what they have. In nonmonogamy, envy is the voice inside your head that talks a lot of smack. You can envy the amount of time people spend together: "She gets to see him twice a week and I only get to see him once a month." You can envy a couple's connection: "They have a much stronger bond than she and I do." You can envy their relationship dynamic: "I wish I were his primary partner." You can envy a partner's partner: "She is so much more experienced and poised than I am."

Competitiveness can be a part of envy; this comes up especially in couples where one partner has numerous sex mates and the other doesn't. In some instances, it's a matter of timing and logistics. In others, it's a personality thing: one partner is a charismatic social butterfly who seems to attract lovers like nectar, while the other is shy, reserved, takes longer to establish a connection with someone. Envious thoughts can be fleeting, easily acknowledged and dismissed, or they can be obsessive and overwhelming.

When you are content with who you are and feel secure and satisfied in your relationship, it greatly lessens your envy of others. Work on yourself and your relationships rather than being preoccupied by others around you. Value yourself and be grateful for what you have. If you see something in someone else or in their relationship that you really want, and it is attainable, take steps to get it by changing something about yourself or your relationship. Otherwise, it's best to work on your own self-worth and insecurities to lessen or eliminate the envy.

Insecurity

Insecurity or low self-esteem is intertwined with envy and is at the heart of most jealous feelings. It may take the form of self-doubt, self-judgment, constant comparisons to others (especially to a partner's other partners), or feeling not good enough. If you don't feel good about yourself or about your relationship, someone new entering the picture raises all kinds of doubt and insecurity. Like envy, insecurity is the voice inside your head that taunts you: "She's prettier than me. His sexual appetite is bigger than mine. She's more my partner's type. He has more in common with my husband."

Insecurity comes from many sources and manifests itself in many ways; it's a complex problem to deal with. First, you must truly believe in the possibility of an open relationship—that you can have sex with more than one person or love multiple people at the same time. If you don't, you will *always* see other people and other relationships as infringing on and threatening to yours. Next, you need to separate yourself from your partner's desires and relationships that don't involve you, because they are truly *not about you*. The beauty of exploring relationship possibilities beyond monogamy is that we are free to explore different desires, fantasies, and interpersonal dynamics with other people. If your partner picks a lover who is into spanking and very good at it, it doesn't mean he wishes *you* were a spanking aficionado and expert. That relationship does not represent a deficit in your relationship, it is not a comment on your relationship, and it is not about replacing you.

> *I find myself asking myself, when I'm feeling jealous, Do I have such little faith in myself and my value as a person that I think I could be so easily replaced? Again, it comes around to forcing myself to take care of myself. When I solidly believe in my worth as a person, there is room for others in my partners' lives.*
> —Elizabeth

If you don't feel secure in who you are and in the strength of your relationship, examine why that is. For instance, you may be experiencing your own issues of inadequacy or fear of abandonment. If that's the case, you need to do some work to tackle the root of those issues. Working on one's self-esteem is not an overnight project; it takes a tremendous amount of time, dedication, and perseverance. That said, there is a difference between feeling unlovable (you're not good enough, you don't deserve love) and feeling unloved. Your sense of insecurity could stem from not getting something you need from your partner to feel secure. Perhaps he hasn't been affectionate enough or hasn't made an effort to set aside quality time for you. In that case, you need to sit down with your partner and talk about it.

Sometimes our insecurity is fueled by our imagination: we imagine a partner's new partner to be the most perfect human being in the world. This kind of thinking—based not on facts, but on our worst fears—can often be corrected with a simple reality check: meet the partner. When you meet her in the flesh, it's harder to irrationally suspect, dislike, or demonize her or to put her on a pedestal.

If it's not you but your partner who feels insecure, your number one job is to provide reassurance. We all need to be reassured that our partners love us, are committed to us, and are not going to leave us. Reassurance is especially important in nonmonogamous relationships, because they can spark feelings of insecurity in us so easily. Clearly articulate to your partner that you love and cherish her and aren't trying to replace her.

Possessiveness

Sometimes you can experience jealousy as a desire to possess or control your partner. If you're the type who considers your lovers *yours* and you don't like to share them, you may find open relationships especially challenging. At the core of possessiveness are two beliefs:

that a person can be a possession, and that there is not enough of him to be shared. In other words, how dare you take something that belongs to me, or take his time away from me? Both beliefs are problematic: people cannot be owned, and being someone's partner doesn't mean you're entitled to all of their time, energy, and love.

The opposite of possessiveness is generosity. As Raven Kaldera writes,

> If you are being generous, it means you have enough to share. You can give plenty away and still not be impoverished. It's that feeling of pure abundance when you know you've got enough of whatever it is that you can give it out by the handfuls and still be knee-deep in it.[3]

Many people in polyamorous relationships would concur. Theo is a 46-year-old man from Connecticut who's been polyamorous for almost 20 years and currently lives with his primary partner of seven years:

> *What makes it easy to share is when we're feeling so full of love and acknowledgment from each other that we're overflowing… When she's acknowledging me and I her and we're really appreciating each other, things heat up. When we're not having a great time together, we're not feeling full of each other, I've been away for three weeks traveling for work, or we're squabbling, then we're not full and we don't feel so great. Then having her be with someone else or having me be with someone else [can] be hard. It's a hell of a lot better when we're full of each other and sexy with each other. Then it's a lot more fun to include the rest.*

Kaldera is articulating a world view, while Theo is speaking of one's perception at a given moment. I think possessiveness and generosity can depend on either impulse—or both. If you are territorial and don't like to share, it's probably difficult for you to share your partners.

Possessive people can learn to separate themselves from their partners and see their partners as independent, freethinking individuals. Perhaps your generosity depends on the particular circumstance: when you feel content and secure and all is well, you're thrilled to share your partner, but when you're feeling shaky or disconnected, you're more apt to experience fear and doubt. One interviewee has another way to deal with possessiveness; Jimmy is a leatherman from Pittsburgh who has several Dominant/submissive relationships: "Being polyamorous doesn't mean I don't get jealous. I'm a very possessive person... Poly's good for me because then I can have more people. I can say 'mine' about a lot of people...mine, mine, mine. I can possess many."

Feeling Excluded

When some people say they feel jealous, what they deeply feel is left out. They wish they could be included in a partner's activities and adventures. For example: I'm jealous that my lover Jenny gets to go to a sex party and I have to stay home and study. Or Jenny's partner takes her on lavish vacations, and I wish I could go with them and see all the exotic places they see. Or Jenny is going to meet all sorts of cool people at the polyamory conference this weekend, and I wish I could be there, too.

Sometimes, the desire to be included can be fulfilled: you can make an agreement with a partner always to have sex or dates with other people together. In other cases, where being included is not possible, realistic, or desirable, you can find ways to manage the feelings. One fairly simple solution: when your partner goes on a date, make plans to do something with a friend; keeping busy is better than sitting home alone, wallowing in jealousy. Or ask your partner to plan dates on a night when you have a class or regular activity. For some people, hearing the details of a partner's dates can be another way for them to feel included and in the loop. While these strategies can help you cope with the feeling, to get to the heart of the matter, work on this goal: you must strongly believe in and support your partner having physical and emotional space to experience things without you.

Coping with Jealousy

If you are the person who feels jealous, the first step is to *let yourself feel jealous*. Even if you know, intellectually, that your emotion is irrational, you can still experience jealousy as real, visceral, and overwhelming. So let yourself feel it—validate and own the feeling. Don't criticize yourself or pile shame and judgment on top of it—that will just make you feel worse.

Remember, too, that jealousy can be a learned reaction, one we see represented and reinforced all around us. Remind yourself that you may be reacting unconsciously in a way you think you should react. Ed, who lives in a triad with his wife and co-husband, says:

> When I find disagreeable emotions surfacing, I take some time to think about it. I rarely react right away to emotions. I'll double-check my beliefs, and see if the emotion is based on values I consciously choose, or if it is a remnant of my earlier social training. For example, one time at a party I saw Leslie smooching and snuggling with her new boyfriend, and I felt a bit jealous. According to the books I've read and the movies I've seen, I should fly into a jealous rage or make some sort of scene. I'm very much in uncharted territory on how to behave; I haven't seen good polyamorous reactions portrayed in movies and such. At the time, I stepped out of the party, and went through my values: Do I think Leslie has complete control over her time, energy and affections? Yes. Do I trust that Leslie still loves me? Yes. And so on, until I concluded that my feelings were coming from a value system I have consciously refused.

When you feel any kind of jealousy, first ask yourself what's underneath the feeling. Do you feel left out, possessive, envious? Are you comparing yourself to someone else? Do you feel threatened, disrespected, angry? Did something specific happen to trigger your jealousy? Remember that we often can't predict whether something will bother us until it happens and we get upset.

Next, seek support from friends, family, or a therapist. Your support system will help you assess the reality of the situation as well as any suspicions or fears you may have. People who love and support you can help you see that your partner's new partner is not the best thing since sliced bread (or whatever it is you've made them out to be) and reassure you that your relationship is solid. Finally, figure out what you need to feel better; it may be time to yourself, reassurance from your partner, or a commitment for some quality time.

I try very hard to accept and cradle my feelings, while recognizing that they are sometimes about issues and relationships that aren't the ones at hand. —Hailey

It's my duty to deal with my negative emotions in a self-caring way and not to dump on my partner, and he returns the favor. —Shari

Some people discover that their jealousy has nothing to do with a partner's actions, so they choose to work on the feelings themselves. Self-care, which is simply being able to soothe, reassure, and take care of yourself when you're feeling bad, is a necessary skill when struggling with jealousy. This can include meditating, writing in a journal, spending time with friends, exercising, doing something creative, or pampering yourself. Other people need to share their feelings with a partner in order to help resolve them. When expressing yourself, take responsibility for how you feel. Your feelings are yours, so don't project them on the other person. A helpful way to do this is a tool of

Nonviolent Communication often referred to as using "I" language. Using "I" language helps you to own your feelings and not blame others for them. Here are some examples:

- "Your taking Sara to the zoo hurt my feelings." (I put the blame on you.)
  "I felt hurt when you took Sara to the zoo instead of me." (This is how I feel.)
- "Your make-out session with Louis at the party made me angry." (I put the blame on you.)
  "I felt angry when I saw you making out with Louis." (This is how I feel.)

After sharing how you feel, talk about what you need to feel better. Keep in mind that your feelings may prompt a new agreement or rule between you, one which can help prevent or alleviate jealousy in the future. For example: The next time we go to a party and hook up with someone, let's not have intercourse with her. Or: I'd prefer it if you didn't take your other partner to the knitting circle, since lots of my friends go to it.

> If I feel that my partner is doing something that makes me feel unduly insecure, I'll ask them not to do it as long as it's not something that'll infringe too much on their life, like "Sweetie, could you not keep telling me how hot X is or, if you do, could you mix it with equal praise of me?" instead of "Could you not speak to X anymore?" —Coraline

If your partner tells you she's feeling jealous, your responsibility is to listen without judgment. Validate her feelings even if you don't understand them. Be present and available to process with her. If your partner comes to you feeling bad, never reject her by saying, "I followed our agreement. This is your problem, deal with it yourself." Some people believe in this "tough love" approach, holding each person solely responsible for his or her own feelings. While I believe we are responsible for our own feelings, I don't think this means leaving your partner stranded to process on his own. You don't need to take the blame for how someone else feels or take his issues on as your own. However, if you are in a relationship, you've made a commitment; you should invest in working on, healing, or fixing the problem in whatever way you can. In addition to listening, reassure your jealous partner about your desire, love, and commitment. Give her a reality check if you feel her fears are unreasonable.

We address each other's feelings with care, urgency, and without judgment. Many assume that one person is isolated in feeling jealous, is responsible for feeling that way, and should take care of these emotions alone. We see that feelings belong to the relationship, thus we both are responsible for the care, resolution, and nurture of them. —Claire

Fear of Abandonment

Behind jealousy, and the insecurity that fuels it, is fear. Usually the fear concerns a change in the relationship or its end. Fear of the unknown is a very powerful emotion. You fear that your partner will fall in love with someone else—which may or may not be on the table as an option depending on your nonmonogamy agreement. You fear that your lover will leave you for this other person. You fear that your role as primary will be taken over. You fear you'll be a failure because the relationship failed. You may even fear that you will be alone forever.

The first tool you need to calm this fear is a reality check: look at the situation rationally, with reassurance from your partner and friends, and see that your relationship is not going to end anytime soon. Don't let those little demon voices in your head tell you otherwise. Look at your fear as a symptom of distrust: if you trusted your partner and your relationship, then you'd know it wasn't in danger. If your partner has not given you any reason *not* to trust her, then the fear is exposed as irrational. But remind your partner not to neglect you as she pursues a new fling or relationship, because ignoring you will only feed into your fear. Ginger says, "I think a lot of this for me is a hangover from monogamous life, where getting a new love means dumping the old one. But that's not what polyamory is about."

One of the best ways to deal with a fear of abandonment is to look it straight in the eye. Embrace the notion that your relationship might be about to end (which, remember, it most likely isn't), that any relationship can end at any point, and *you will go on.* It will be painful, horrible, awful, but you will survive. If it ends, it doesn't mean you've failed.

If you make peace with your worst fear coming true, it can't continue to have a powerful hold on you. And make no mistake: the fear of abandonment is a powerful one, usually with roots in a childhood experience of traumatic loss; it takes time and hard work to overcome, and it doesn't go away just by wishing it will. If you feel that this fear is a driving force in your life, causing you excessive worry or leading you to compromise your own needs, then I recommend counseling.

Resentment

People feel resentment when they believe someone has hurt or wronged them; resentment is a kind of anger that usually stays unresolved. People grow angry when their needs are not met, when they feel unappreciated, or when a partner does something they feel is hurtful. Resentment often comes up in open relationships when one partner goes along with some behavior to make the other happy: these are the times when you say yes to a partner's request for a sexual encounter or a new partner but your heart screams no. You should never give something your blessing if you have reservations about it. When you don't honor your feelings and instincts, when you don't verbalize what you want and need, when you keep silent so you don't rock the boat, it's only a matter of time before you feel bad. Unexpressed anger and resentment can only lead to a breakdown in communication, distance between partners, and a pileup of negative emotions.

Letting things build up over time can lead to painful emotional explosions. The resentful partner has reached his limit and lets loose days or weeks or years of hurt and anger; usually the other partner feels blindsided, since he's hearing the information for the first time. We can't expect our partners to read our minds. The key to avoiding resentment is to express your feelings, even if they are difficult to talk about, like anger, hurt, or betrayal. Even if you know the feelings are irrational, you must still honor them and communicate them.

PROFILE: FIONA AND SAM

> *"We continually work at figuring out what is good*
> *for the relationship."*

FIONA, 36, IS A SPECIAL EDUCATION TEACHER and university instructor. Sam is a 32-year-old student in social work and education. They have been together in a polyamorous relationship for five years and live in Brooklyn.

What are the rules, boundaries, and limits in your relationship?

Fiona: I think what has been successful for us is to conceptualize things differently. We don't "negotiate" or focus on limits or boundaries. That is not to say anything goes! Rather, we work continually to create our relationship and how we relate to others. This is something we have had a lot of help with, particularly from our therapist. We continually work at figuring out what is good for the relationship. So, rather then set it up as my needs versus yours, my desires versus yours, my boundaries versus yours, we try to decide what the relationship can handle at any given time. For example, we have some working guidelines. If you are out at a bar or party, you can make out or fool around with other people. But if we have a fight when one person is leaving the house, or one person is in a bad way for whatever reason, then it is not a *rule* but it is the culture of our relationship for the person who is going out to decide it is probably not a good night to hook up at the bar.

How do you deal with negative feelings like jealousy, possessiveness, insecurity, anger, resentment?

Fiona: Sometimes I talk to a friend, change the channel of my mind, or use some other tactic to remind myself that it is no big deal and that I have a million more important things to worry about. Other times I take anger and upset and frustration to be a sign that things are not working for me, that I don't like how I am being treated or what we have agreed to. Then I get help by talking to other people and talking to Sam.

Sam: I have been amazed at how much *less* jealous and possessive I have felt within this relationship than in the past. Somehow having it out there that *of course* we are both attracted to other people has been a huge relief—and means that I trust it a lot more when Fiona says she wants to be with me—because I know she is being honest, and can have those other attractions and experiences at the same time. An exception would be our relationship with Brooke, when I really wasn't able or willing to put my relationship with Fiona ahead of my immediate, selfish wants... That was a very painful time. All those feelings came into play during that time...and I don't think any of us dealt with them very lovingly or effectively, perhaps most especially me.

Tell me more about the relationship with Brooke.

Fiona: Sam and I had a joint girlfriend for six months.

Sam: My connection with Brooke was really intense. She and I got together first and were involved to a certain degree separately from Fiona. Then we stopped that because...our connection wasn't okay for Fiona's and my relationship, it wasn't working. Then, Brooke and Fiona went out one night and kissed...it was really exciting. These two very intense relationships. They had a connection that was sometimes really hot and awesome and fun, but there were also lots of ways that they didn't completely mesh.

Fiona: It was beautiful at moments. Fun. Hot. Sex. Magical. Oh-so-intimate. At times it was exactly why I wanted to be poly. I saw up close the intense and wonderful connection between Brooke and Sam. The emotion in our threesome and in our respective twosomes ran really, really high—from the extremely close, connected, and wonderful to the crazed, angry, and upset. I was into the ideal of a threesome and into the ideal of supporting Sam to pursue this relationship with someone he had a really deep connection with. But, day to day, it turned out I wanted to have just...[a] Sam-and-I twosome. I think I made a big mistake in that I underestimated how important our shared home, shared evenings, shared time, just the two of us was. So time and again, when Brooke said, "Hey, I am in the neighborhood, can I come over?" I said yes, but for me it ended up being too much, too fast, and ultimately not what I wanted or could handle—even though I adored her and believed in the idea of it all so strongly.

Sam: We were trying to do something challenging—really sustain a threesome relationship—and I think none of us were quite sure what we really wanted from it or from each other. We really didn't have the support we needed to figure it out. Even friends of ours who were into the idea of being poly couldn't really handle it or didn't know what to make of what we were doing. I was so aware that we were really making things up each moment... This is one of the things I *love* about being poly—that it challenges me to be creative and to live as authentically as possible, but it is incredibly difficult, especially when emotions run high.

Fiona: So, it just became a mess. We were all really awful to one another. We said a lot of mean things and just struggled for months. Ultimately, Brooke ended it, and one of my most intimate evenings with her was when she told me she realized she needed to move on, that she wanted a partner and kids, and being with us was not a move toward that. It was so hard for me to let go. I wanted her in our lives. I held out a fantasy that she would move in with us. But I think it just wasn't right for any of us, despite our love and attraction.

Looking back on it now, what did you learn from it?

Sam: One lesson I learned was to be much more cautious about checking in about what we want out of [a new relationship]. [Now] I feel much more committed to working and creatively building my relationship with Fiona and to have whatever else happens be a part of that, whether we do it separately or together.

Fiona: I was able to realize how important my relationship with Sam was and that I really didn't want to completely share it with a third person. At the time, I didn't appreciate enough what we had. I was trying to be the party girl and go with the flow. One thing I have learned is to be continually assessing my life and the relationships I have created. Do I like them? Am I happy? Is this working? Is it what I want? To be in the process of my life with people and deciding together what makes sense.

For you, what is the most fundamental element of creating and sustaining a positive poly relationship?

Fiona: Be on the side of the relationship. This is something we learned from our therapist. She has asked us, in different ways over time, Who is going to be on the side of the relationship? After much hard work, we have adopted that. I think we are both now less concerned with "getting" (as in getting what we each need) and more focused on what would be good or growthful for our relationship.

Sam: I have been, within relationships over the years, both cheated on and a cheat, both incredibly jealous/possessive and desperately restless for new hookups. Something about polyamory, at least in the way that Fiona and I do it together, has supported me to more fully embrace Fiona and our relationship and, at the same time, more fully trust, let go, take risks, make new connections... Fiona and I have a strong, loving sexual and emotional connection that continues to grow deeper and more exciting through the years...and part of that is supporting each other to continue to be attracted to and connect with other people, have new experiences, find new passions.

Chapter 13

Compersion

THE WORD *COMPERSION* was coined by members of the Kerista Commune as part of their philosophy of multipartner polyfidelitous relationships. Keristans originally defined compersion as "the opposite of jealousy, positive feelings about your partner's other intimacies." Others have expanded upon the concept; here are some additional definitions:

> taking pleasure or joy in the action of your partner engaging in a similar romantic or sexual relationship with another person. —Urban Dictionary[1]

> the feeling of taking joy in the joy that others you love share among themselves, especially taking joy in the knowledge that your beloveds are expressing their love for one another. —Polyamory Society[2]

> the positive feelings one gets when a lover is enjoying another relationship. Sometimes called the opposite or flip side of jealousy. May coexist with "jealous" feelings. —Poly Oz[3]

an emotional state where your insecurities are so low, your trust so high, and your value in the happiness of your partner(s) so far beyond your own baggage, that seeing them have good relationships with over lovers inspires nothing but joy and contentment in you. —*Pagan Polyamory*[4]

Each definition varies slightly, but the general idea is that compersion is taking joy in your partner's pleasure or happiness with another partner. Compersion is a much-used concept among polyamorous people, and many nonmonogamous people believe it is one of the cornerstones of open relationships. Some would go so far as to say that you cannot succeed without it. I think it's more complicated than that.

One form of compersion, which I call erotic compersion, can be achieved when you enjoy or get turned on by watching your partner have sex with someone else. Many nonmonogamous people who have threesomes, group sex, public sex, or semipublic sex are aroused by seeing a partner with someone else, whether they are participating or not. Claire and her partner almost always play with other people together. She says, "Seeing him in ecstasy, seeing someone else with him in ecstasy, I feel it... I feel like I'm very much a part of it. It's not intellectual and it's not emotional...it's visceral."

When Dahlia and her partner arranged a play date with another person, she experienced erotic compersion in a dramatic way, and it was a breakthrough for her:

When this person was fucking my partner in the ass, I lay down on the other bed and began to masturbate with the Magic Wand. I got so turned on watching my spouse getting fucked that I had one of the mightiest orgasms I've ever had. This may seem commonplace, but one needs to know a little background first. I didn't start masturbating until I was 26, as I grew up in a fundamentalist Christian home, and the only kind of sex that was allowed was when one got married to a member of the "opposite" sex and that person had to be a born-again Christian. Masturbation was considered "of the devil," and only served to promote lust and selfishness... Even though I finally started masturbating at my late age, I had never masturbated in front of anyone before. It even took some time for me to be able to do it in front of my spouse. So, the fact that I had this huge orgasm in front of an almost complete stranger was very exciting for me.

Some people who experience erotic compersion don't even need to be present to be turned on. For example:

When my husband and I were first dating and he was on a date with someone else, I knew their intention was to have sex. I was alone that night. So I was kind of sitting around with this icky feeling like, Oh my god, what does this mean, maybe I'm not pretty enough—all those insidious things—and I just started imagining the two of them together. It was so incredibly beautiful, it was a turn-on. So I brought out my Hitachi [vibrator] and had these amazing orgasms thinking about them having sex together. Somehow eroticizing it took away the ickiness and replaced it with excitement. —Ruby Grace

While erotic compersion can be powerful, deriving pleasure from your partner's other relationships goes deeper for most people. In an ideal world, when your partner is happy, you're happy, even if you have done nothing to provoke her happiness. But this may be easier said than done for folks who wrestle with jealousy. People work hard to tolerate and support their partner's other relationships. It's one thing to accept that your partner has other lovers or partners; it's another to take joy in them. The gap between acceptance and joy can be wide.

Serena Anderlini-D'Onofrio writes that compersion is, in part, "the ability to turn jealousy's negative feelings into acceptance of, and vicarious enjoyment for, a lover's joy."[5] I appreciate that she treats acceptance as a skill that can be learned rather than as a static state of mind. It is not a skill that most of us are taught or that is encouraged by our culture—a culture much more given to encouraging and reinforcing jealousy and competitiveness.

For some, compersion can be learned, and like anything else, it takes patience and practice. We are taught that jealousy is innate, natural, instinctual; in fact, people who don't get jealous are considered strange or in denial. Jealousy is a learned behavior. The first step to achieving compersion is to work on unlearning jealousy—letting go of feelings of insecurity, possessiveness, and fear. You're striving for a shift in consciousness. One way to begin is to think back to a time when you felt excited for your partner, not threatened, when he revealed a crush. For example, Sam says:

> *Fiona supported, pushed, and challenged me to hook up with this trans boy I had a big crush on…it was a new experience for me, to get together with a boy as a boy (instead of as the heterosexual girl I had tried to be as a teenager). I was very nervous and hesitant about it. He and I did end up hooking up that night and on several other occasions. Fiona and I both had a ton of fun with the whole thing. It was the first time I had ever really acted on my attraction to someone besides my partner in a truly honest, open, poly sort of way…It definitely felt overwhelming and surprising, confusing, and absolutely wonderful that Fiona was so supportive and into it—and often right in the next room when we were hooking up.*

In this case, Fiona felt so positively about her partner Sam's crush that she actually helped facilitate the hookup. Others have described similar times when they felt they were in cahoots with their partner to make something happen, even if both of them weren't involved in it. To conceptualize it another way: if you love your partner and are dedicated to her growth, anything that enriches her life or encourages growth should please you. It can even benefit you: when a partner is involved with someone else, they explore, learn, and change, and that can make your relationship better.

> *I enjoy seeing my other partners happy with someone else. It makes me happy to see them being happy and made happy by someone. It also strengthens our relationship because they bring that love and happiness back to us.* —Marcus

In his essay on compersion, Eric Francis argues that we must bring all our deepest fears out in the open and confront them:

> It is true that if one's lover has sex with another person, or even gets close to another person, they may choose to be with that person and not you. And this is a possibility we have to face no matter what. Living the way of compersion brings this to the surface, where we can see it and work with it… Resentment, anger, fear of abandonment, and the rest—all needs to come up in order to give the relationship a chance to have life. Swept under the rug, these things are far more damaging… Compersion takes us to the next realm beyond. It is about being with and appreciating our partners for their desires, dreams, wishes, and their personal journey to self-love. It's about being real, and having relationships as real people.[6]

Francis believes that jealousy is the fear of loss, and in those terms, compersion is a kind of fearlessness, or at least embracing the fear and not letting it drive your decisions. James is a 57-year-old Latino man who teaches Tantra. He's in an open relationship with his partner and strongly believes that embracing his fear helps him bring authenticity to his life and relationship:

> *Just think how alive you live every day, knowing the possibility [of the relationship ending] is there and that edge is there. Even though*

it is the hardest thing, to me, it's the most real way to live with somebody. You're really creating that relationship every single second. And if something comes up that's going to change that relationship, you both have to look at it and say, "Am I willing to focus on your happiness and your evolution even if it means losing you?" Yeah. Absolutely. Why would I want you to stay with me if you really have lust and passion for somebody else? Go for it, don't waste time. Even though security is the hardest thing that you're always dealing with—because you can lose everything that's real to you in a second—I wouldn't trade it for the world.

Part of achieving compersion is letting go of any perceived control we have over our partners. When you do this, you give your partner the freedom and support to grow and change in whatever ways he needs. If you are new to open relationships, you should not expect to master compersion right away. I do not believe that experiencing compersion is *necessary* to a functional open relationship in the way that other values, beliefs, and practices are, but it is bound to enhance your relationship. The closer you come to embracing the spirit of compersion, the better you are at managing jealousy, letting go of possessiveness, and feeling positive about all your partner's relationships—even the ones you're not a part of.

PROFILE: LUKE AND ILANA

"We develop other intimate relationships that nourish us and help us develop along our growth path."

ILANA AND LUKE have been married for almost 20 years. She's 47, he's fiftysomething, and they both work as consultants. They live in the Deep South.

When you first got together, was the relationship open from day one?

Luke: About a year after my divorce, Ilana and I started dating. She was dating other people at the time. She didn't want to change that, so from the get-go it was a nonmonogamous relationship, which was quite different from my model. I was raised Catholic, had had a good Catholic marriage. Infidelity was right up there with murder as a grievous sin.

What was that transition to nonmonogamy like for you?

Luke: It was a little challenging at first... Within the first year of our being together and having outside relationships, we just worked into what felt right, what felt comfortable, what was allowable, how deep we could go in other relationships. We were just sort of defining all that along the way. Ilana is my primary. I want and need a primary in my life. I view marriage as the way to make this sacred commitment with one. I've very rarely not been in some kind of serious relationship where I was investing all my emotional energy...having that kind of commitment, partnership, is just somehow in touch with my being... When I have other relationships or fall in love, it's totally different. I don't have conversations about our retirement, how to manage our money, what kind of furniture do we want to buy... Having all that other stuff—how you met, how you spend your life, kids, how you're gonna grow old, dreams... I really feel much more complete and centered and whole when I have one person with whom I can share that.

Ilana: I love having a committed life partner, though initially I wasn't sure I ever was interested in "marriage." Early on, after five years of living together and owning a house, my husband really needed and wanted to be married. I decided I wanted him as a life partner, so marriage made sense at the time. We hadn't considered whether we were poly or open...we just communicated our needs and values and accommodated each other in ways that made things work. In some ways, now, our marriage is problematic in the traditional culture we live in. Our marriage is quite different from what most people assume "marriage" means—in this part of the country at least.

Luke: I can elaborate on that a bit: people feel they have their own set of rules and definitions as to what marriage is. If we do something outside that, it can raise eyebrows. If I agree to lunch with a woman, just purely as a friendship, not even a relationship, per se, that seems outside the realm of acceptable behavior for a lot of people here. They project their definition of marriage on us, and if we live outside their definition, it raises flags, questions, issues, gossip, and sometimes outright condemnation.

How is it for you to be in such a nontraditional relationship in the Bible Belt?

Luke: We would not have an outside relationship here in town, in part [because] if someone went off the deep end, caused a lot of problems, we wouldn't know how to deal with it logistically. So, most of our relationships have really been the result of travels. We both travel a lot, for business and pleasure, so we'd find relationships in places we'd travel to frequently rather than here at home. In terms of being in the Deep South and living openly and honestly who we are, it's really a challenge.

Do you have other partners right now?

Luke: For the last five years or so, we've been involved with two other couples, and…it's grown into these deep, loving relationships. We anticipate these being lifelong friends, an ongoing part of the fabric of our lives, more the warp than the weave, and that's been a new experience for us that we've really been enjoying. I don't know if that's unique to us, or couples with couples share some common issues that couples with singles don't share.

Ilana: It's been valuable being able to travel together, share about relationship issues together. I will forever be grateful for the gifts from these relationships: personal growth and awareness as well as ecstasy, joy, sacred sexual spiritual transcendence, contentment, deep love, and connection—and a deeper, stronger relationship with my primary partner/husband. There's tremendous richness and growth in intimate relationships. Partners can be on our growth edge. And as that edge moves and changes over time, we develop other intimate relationships that nourish us and help us develop along our growth path.

Luke: I think outside relationships have tremendous potential for personal growth, both individually and for your primary relationship. But this is only true if you have a primary relationship that is safe and secure and flourishing. There's so much scripting we've grown up with that really just needs to be thrown out. When you get involved with somebody, learning who they are and growing this intimate relationship, if the possibility of sex is on the table, you put up all these filters—can I say this, can I do that, can we spend this kind of time together. There's just all these filters and structures. Most of the time you don't even know what they are because you're running on different playbooks, different rules. Once you take the sex off the table and say, "This relationship can be absolutely anything," then the relationship will be anything that the magic and the chemistry of two people can create. It is just so much richer and deeper, and you can get there so much more quickly because you're not fumbling through restrictions, prejudices, rules. We've both discovered how rich relationships can be when you take the rules off the table and let them evolve into whatever they need to be.

Chapter 14

Common Challenges and Problems

THE JEALOUSY AND OTHER FEELINGS discussed in Chapter 12 can cause angst, hurt, conflict, and drama between partners. Such intense emotions can cause problems and fuel arguments in any relationship, not just an open one. People in nonmonogamous relationships face all the issues that monogamous people do; however, certain problems are specific to nonmonogamy or seem to crop up more frequently when a relationship is open. These include complications from "new relationship energy"; time management issues; miscommunication; the violation of rules and agreements; coping with change; coming out and dealing with reactions from loved ones. In this chapter, we explore all but the last two. Change is the subject of Chapter 15, Opening Up Again: When Something Changes; dealing with loved ones is covered in Chapter 16, Coming Out (or Not), Finding Community, Creating Families.

New Relationship Energy (NRE)

When you meet someone you feel a spark with—whether you want to fuck, fall in love, or both—you usually feel a rush of excitement. You're flying high, crushed out, and falling hard. Some social scientists refer to this as a state of *limerence*. The psychologist Dorothy Tennov coined the term in her 1979 book *Love and Limerence: The Experience of Being in Love*. After interviewing 500 people about being in love, she identified a common pattern marked by the following characteristics:

- intrusive thinking about the object of your desire
- acute longing
- dependency of your mood on the person's actions
- inability to react limerently to more than one person at a time
- fear of rejection and shyness around the person
- vivid imagination about the person
- intensification through adversity
- an aching in the chest or stomach when uncertainty is strong
- acute sensitivity to any act, thought, or condition that can be interpreted favorably, and an extraordinary ability to devise or invent "reasonable" explanations for why neutral actions are a sign of hidden passion in the person
- buoyancy (a feeling of walking on air) when reciprocation seems evident
- a general intensity of feeling that leaves other concerns in the background
- a remarkable ability to emphasize what is truly admirable in the person and to avoid dwelling on the negative or render it into another positive attribute.[1]

Tennov's research was limited to the experience of being in love, but feelings of intense desire, lust, and connection can also produce some of the characteristics of limerence.

When you meet someone you like, when your crush is reciprocated, when you first pursue a relationship, you're blissed out. You can't get your mind off him. You're anxious until the next time you see her. You're completely focused on the two of you—it's easy to shut out the rest of the world. When you're together, you can't keep your hands off each other. Research has shown that many of these feelings and behaviors stem from chemical changes in your brain. When you first feel attraction, begin a relationship, and fall in love, levels of dopamine and norepinephrine (natural stimulants) increase in the limbic system; in addition, activity increases in the parts of your brain involved in arousal and pleasure.

When you bundle together the physical (chemical changes in your body) and the emotional and psychological (intense feelings and thoughts), you've got what some people call *new relationship energy* (often referred to as NRE)[2]. The term was coined by Zhahai Stewart in the mid-1980s and has been commonly used by polyamorous people since the 1990s.[3]

NRE is that euphoric state of love or lust in which the world seems to revolve around the new person. It is both wonderful and dangerous. It's wonderful because you feel energized, alive, excited, and thrilled at having found a mutual connection with someone. You want to tell everyone about her; you tend to see all of her positive aspects and none of her flaws. One of the benefits of open relationships is the ability to experience NRE without having to end an existing relationship. How can such wonderful feelings be dangerous for people in open relationships? During this period, your judgment is altered—it's fueled by hormones and desire and clouded by overwhelming feelings of love and lust. Many people report that when a partner is experiencing NRE, they are focused only on themselves and the new partner; they neglect other partners, do callous things, and make rash decisions. NRE can cause grievous heartache to one's partners, and it has been known to break up relationships.

Coping with NRE

Nonmonogamy veterans recognize NRE. They know it's a phase that will eventually pass, and many just ride it out. Even the most experienced among us can feel frustrated when a partner is caught up in the dizzying world of a new fling or relationship. The key to maintaining your sanity is patience. Allow the person who is in NRE the freedom to ride the high, but caution him against making any significant decisions during this period. Remind him that he has other commitments and not to neglect them for this new person. A common conflict occurs when the partner of the person who is head over heels attempts to offer an objective perspective, perhaps expressing concerns about the new person. This partner is grounded, experienced, and can see drama coming from a mile away. The fool for love can't see anything negative and accuses his partner of being jealous and possessive. This is why it's important to know when you're in the midst of an NRE haze. Leslie talks about the dangers of telling a partner about her concerns regarding a new person:

> *[It's difficult to let] a primary partner date someone you suspect is not good for them, for your primary relationship, or [who] might not be poly. [It's difficult to] let them make what you think are relationship mistakes and to express your concerns about these relationships without triggering defensiveness. A person in NRE will greatly defend their new love. Many of us married polys have been in the position of having our concerns dismissed, or being criticized for having them in the first place, only to later have our spouse admit we were right to be concerned. This is hard, because it means you are against a new love of theirs, and that places strain on your primary relationship at a time when they are swimming in strong emotions. The concerned primary has to communicate carefully and as respectfully as possible, and the primary in NRE has to listen without dismissing, criticizing, or assuming it's just their spouse's problem. The concerned spouse also has to greatly self-analyze themselves to make sure their concerns are valid and they are not just acting out of their own insecurities in the face of their partner's strong NRE. It's cloudy, fuzzy, emotional.*

When Violet's partner Ron got involved with someone new, his behavior troubled her, but she decided not to freak out:

Violet: *With Lila, all sorts of new relationship energy was really coming out in a way that hadn't with anybody else I'd ever seen. You were kind of manic. It made me feel a little insecure. You acted differently. It seemed very strange and it was a little threatening. I could tell you were really gaga over this person. I was, at that point, in my denial thing: I don't know what's going on here. I better just leave it alone and do my own thing. And whatever happens, happens.*

Ron: *In fact what I got from you was an amazing amount of support to pursue [the relationship with Lila]. I knew you were feeling fear, but I didn't get demands for reassurance, or promises that nothing bad was going to happen, or anything else. And that allowed that relationship to take its own particular trajectory—into the brick wall. There's a way in which you can imagine pressure from someone else will make things work differently. And in this case the relationship did probably what both Lila and I knew it was going to do, which was to crash and burn.*

In the end, Ron's new relationship was destined to "crash and burn," but Violet's willingness to step back from the situation and be patient, despite her concerns, meant that it didn't cause conflict in their relationship.

If you're the one experiencing NRE, acknowledge that it's happening and be aware of the crazy state you're in. Pay close attention to your existing partners and relationships: be conscious not to neglect them or take them for granted, and be sensitive to how they feel. Channel your newfound burst of love and energy to benefit all your relationships, not just the new one. Don't make significant decisions in the throes of NRE, such as: Let's move in together! I'll lend you $1,000! Let's start a business together! I want to move across the country! Take a deep breath and remember there's plenty of time to make major life changes later. Listen to your loved ones. Remember that you have your head up your ass, so if someone who knows you well and loves you tells you you're acting like a buffoon or headed for trouble, listen.

Raven Kaldera calls NRE the "Shiny New Lover Syndrome" and points out that it can feed right into another's fear of abandonment: "Shiny New Lover Syndrome can generate huge arguments, demands, and conflicts. To the person on the other end, it feels suspiciously like you've left them, even when you're still there."[4] Colin learned this first-hand, though the experience helped strengthen his primary relationship in the end:

> When I was involved in my first poly relationship, the first one outside my marriage, I was really excited about it, and wanting to do lots of crazy and romantic things. I wanted to go camping with [my new partner], for instance. My wife was unhappy that "we never go camping." It was a slow and somewhat painful process of figuring out how our marriage of five years at the time had become static and complacent. I value what we learned, because we have a more active primary relationship now, but it was very uncomfortable to go through.

As in Colin's story, NRE can be an opportunity to revitalize your existing relationships. Feeling excited about life again? Sex drive going through the roof? Reinspired to dust off that guitar and start lessons again? Take some of your newfound energy and inspiration from the new relationship and let it spill over into your existing ones. Rather than get caught up in it, distracted, and focused only on the new person, if you learn how to channel NRE, it can help you improve—rather than jeopardize—all your relationships.

> While you're busy lavishing yourself all over the new partner, which is a marvelous and good and fine and lovely thing, make sure you rub up against your existing partner some too. —Bear

Another thing to be aware of is that NRE is so powerful that some people act compulsively so they can experience it often. Such people are always on the prowl, looking for the hot new thing to keep them constantly in that altered state of bliss. One of my interviewees, Cheryl, called herself an "NRE junkie," and it's certainly possible for people to get hooked on the amazing feelings of NRE. Be aware of the possibility, check your motives for pursuing someone new, and, above all, use common sense.

Time Management

The number one difficulty with nonmonogamy cited by the people I interviewed was time management. You can have an unlimited amount of love, affection, energy, and emotion to give to people, but there are only so many hours in a day. Add to that other obligations like work, school, and children, plus the time and cost to travel for long-distance relationships, and it's a huge challenge in our hectic, fast-paced, over-scheduled world. But spending quality time with your partners is important to nurturing your relationships, so it must be made a priority. What's a busy nonmonogamous person to do?

The first step in good time management is to be realistic: know your priorities and your own limits about what you can and can't do. Assess your commitments, and don't take on another partner if your existing partners feel that they don't see you enough. Don't overcommit yourself, and don't forget to schedule time for yourself *without* any partners. As a general rule, people who are good at open relationships are organized. Seriously, you need a calendar, a PDA, scheduling software—whatever it takes to keep track of your life. Nonmonogamous people must become skilled at scheduling, otherwise it just won't work.

An essential part of scheduling is prioritizing. Decide what is most important to you (I must go to yoga at least two days a week!) and what isn't (I will do pottery only if I have some spare time) and schedule accordingly. Once it's all on the schedule, stick to it as best you can. Your time is valuable, and so is other people's. Respect time limits, keep your dates, and don't cancel at the last minute. That said, you've also got to be flexible: know that things come up unexpectedly and plans must change. Along the same lines, realize when you're feeling overwhelmed, and communicate it. If you're overloaded with stress, you can't have a very good time on a date. If you need some time off, take it.

When you can't see your partner in person, cultivate other forms of communication: we've got everything from cell phones and email to instant messaging and webcams. Some couples even keep up to date with each other by reading (and commenting on) each other's blogs. Or you can embrace the retro cool of writing letters and mailing them. I know people who don't like to talk on the phone and others who hate instant messages. Find a medium that works best for you and use it to stay connected to your sweeties.

If you are in a long-term relationship, especially if you live together, don't take seeing your partner every day for granted. Rushing around to get the children to school and yourselves to work is not quality time. It's important to set aside special time for a date for just the two (or three or four) of you.

Making time for one another has two elements. First, literally, you set aside a specific time to spend together. In their interviews, people in polyfidelitous relationships talked about making time for each two-some—a strategy anyone with multiple partners can adopt. Leslie makes sure she goes on dates with each of her two husbands at least once a week, and sleeps with each twice a week. Like many interviewees, Shawn has an official weekly "date night" with each of his triad partners.

The other element of making time for one another is making that time meaningful. Make it intentional and dedicated. This is not about the number of times per month you see each other, but about the quality of the interaction between you, and the frame of mind you're in. Elizabeth and her primary partner discovered that the key to a successful date night is not seeing (or having intense interactions with) other lovers on that day. She says it helps keep them focused on each other. For Jesse, it's about being aware of his time so he can be present: "I can't reasonably be expected to erase my head space—when I'm with a lover, for instance, and thinking about another. What I can do, however, is be responsible to my needs for alone time, time spent in between lovers, so that when I'm next in a sexual situation I can be [more] present for the person I'm with." Duke says he tries to plan for certain nights with one partner and stick with them. "It means you never have to give anyone the impression of 'deciding' whom you would rather spend your evening with... But also bear in mind that for a while, every time you have to say 'No, I have plans that evening,' it's going to sting someone."

In addition to spending romantic and sexual time together, it's a good idea for people who run a household with multiple partners to hold regular meetings to keep things running smoothly. Use this time to address both practical matters—bills, financial planning, household chores, travel schedules—and emotional ones—unresolved tension, miscommunication, or an issue that needs to be discussed with everyone. Audrey's triad has monthly meetings: "It's a forum where we're all coming to the table willing to accept criticism and discuss whatever's important to everyone else... It is really one of the cornerstones that make our day-to-day relationship successful. Instead of bringing up grievances whenever they just pop into our heads, and everyone's tired and hungry and irritated, this way we all know it's coming, we all prepare for it, and we always have dinner." Ed is in a V triad with his wife, Leslie, and co-husband, Colin: "One of us acts as 'secretary'—we type up the minutes and pass them around, particularly for agreements, as our memories tend to differ and get worse over time."

If you feel that house meetings, planned date nights, and a sleeping schedule are not romantic or spontaneous, I say: get over it. Good time management is a reality that people in open relationships must face.

Miscommunication

Just as good communication is a key component of a successful open relationship, miscommunication is a common cause of conflict. Miscommunication can occur for any number of reasons, even when both parties have good intentions and believe they're on the same page. A common communication pitfall is failing to be specific enough in discussions. People often assume that however they phrase their thoughts, the other person knows exactly what they mean, but this is not always the case. For example, let's say J and K are in a committed relationship and have casual sex mates on the side; they agree that they won't do anything romantic with their fuck buddies. J goes to lunch with one of her flings and tells K about it; K becomes upset: "We said don't do anything romantic, then you go and have lunch with her." J responds, "But it was lunch, not dinner. And it was at a diner!" J thinks of it as a meal between friends and doesn't consider it romantic. The lesson here? Rather than say "I prefer that you don't do romantic things with your sex mates," say "I prefer that you don't have meals or go to movies or the theater with your sex mates."

Becca's primary partner told her it was okay for her to play with other people at BDSM clubs, but when she did and he saw caning marks on her butt, he wasn't happy. "It was one of those 'Go—I am totally okay with it'... [Then] he had a hugely negative reaction to seeing physical evidence of someone else's...um...fun." They made an agreement that she could play with others as long as she didn't come home with marks on her body.

Ginger and her husband, who are kinky and polyamorous, recently faced a huge challenge when Ginger wanted to have a male partner, which caught her husband completely off guard. Ginger says:

Before my husband and I ever met in person or played, I completed a BDSM checklist where you check off likes and dislikes. I think you should have the same kind of conversation early on about poly. Had I filled out a checklist for poly that included "interested in relationships with other men," I probably would have checked Yes. If there was "interested in falling in love with other men," I probably would have checked Yes, or Maybe. Whereas, in his mind, that was never going to come up... There's a lot of serious negotiation in BDSM that's kind of formal and maybe we could do with a little more of that around relationships... Spend a little time talking about what all the possibilities could be in the relationship. I wish we had done that.

Ginger raises a good point about the importance of being specific about not only what you want but *what you may want* down the road. As BDSM practitioners, they were clear and detailed in negotiating what they wanted, but as practitioners of polyamory, they were not.

Miscommunication can also come up when one person acts on an assumption about how the other person will react. It's important to listen to your partner's point of view and act on the information you have. Sometimes, when you don't have enough information, or just out of habit, you make a decision about your partner based on *you*: This is what I would do or this wouldn't hurt my feelings or this would totally be okay with me, so it will be okay with my partner. It's common to assume that the people we love share our values, ideas, expectations, and boundaries. In fact, they often do, but on a specific point your partner may feel quite differently than you. People can get into lots of trouble when they take action based on their own perspective rather than asking for their partner's.

For example, Elizabeth and her secondary partner were having some problems in their relationship and their sex life. They spent an intense weekend together during which they had sex, reconnected, and worked out some of their issues:

Spending three full days with each other alone was a big deal. This was the first time we had to spend with each other uninterrupted in a long time. She had a new lover and I was feeling really insecure about our relationship. We had a wonderful three days. When we parted, I was feeling hopeful and optimistic about our relationship. The night I left her, she went and spent a nonsexual overnight with her new lover. From my lover's perspective, her new lover and I were separate people; one didn't affect the other. She felt we were on good, solid footing after three great days together, and she didn't owe me any additional negotiation. So she was deeply upset that I would undermine the great weekend we had with unfounded insecurity about another person. I, on the other hand, was deeply hurt that she would bed-hop like she did. I felt it was disrespectful to me and undermined all the progress we made in those three days.

Elizabeth's conflict represents what happens when two people see a situation differently: she saw her partner's bed-hopping as disrespectful and callous, whereas her partner saw it as perfectly reasonable based on their agreements.

Elizabeth's problem raises the issue of what I call "the challenge of the gray area." The challenge of the gray area arises when you are faced with a situation that isn't specifically covered by your current agreement; the scenario falls in a gray area. Let's call two male partners C and D. C and D are nonmonogamous and both are serious about not hooking up with people they might know in common in their daily lives. They agree that they won't have affairs with any guys either of them works with. At a party, C meets the brother of a co-worker of D; the brother sometimes does temp work at D's office. C has a dilemma: is the brother off limits or not? The easy solution to a situation like this is simply to ask your partner, but sometimes that's not possible. It's good to have a "contingency plan" for these gray areas. For example: If you're not sure, just don't do it. Or: If you're not sure, use your best judgment and we'll deal with it. Or: If the person is not on an explicit list of people you may not fuck, then go for it.

Callie and Samira encounter problems when they go out to parties without having set clear boundaries about flirting, making out, or picking up others. On the one hand, they don't want to impose a rule such as *No flirting or picking anybody up, ever, while we're there*; that feels too restrictive. On the other hand, Samira does not want it to be a free-for-all. For her, it's simply about respecting the person you come to the party with. She might say, "Could you get that person's number, rather than go make out with them right now?" In the past, when Samira has requested that they not do anything with other people at parties, Callie has accused her of wanting to be monogamous, and it has caused a fight. For Samira, the happy medium would be for the two to "check in a lot" because she recognizes that hard and fast rules don't always work in an unpredictable situation. Without clear boundaries, though, these two continue to have misunderstandings, hurt feelings, and arguments.

Agreement Violation

When people negotiate their needs, desires, and limits, the negotiation culminates in some sort of agreement. It may be verbal or written, brief or detailed, but an understanding has been reached. Agreements are an important part of open relationships. They help to clarify what partners need, want, and expect from one another. They give people a sense of security, reassurance, and commitment in the relationship. One of the most difficult things for people in open relationships to deal with is a partner violating an agreement. This can be especially devastating because of the work you put into the negotiation: you pondered your wants and your boundaries, clearly articulated them, discussed them, and agreed on certain rules or guidelines, only to have them violated.

Imagine that it's your birthday. You haven't told anyone, so you don't get any gifts, and you just feel a little blue. Now imagine that you told your friends it was your birthday, sent them a detailed wish list, and you still didn't get any gifts. You're devastated. When we are clear about our desires and we express them to others, it raises our expectations. Similarly, when someone agrees to a rule or boundary, we expect them to keep their word.

Not all agreement violations have equal weight. They can run the gamut from "You were supposed to call me once a day while you were out of town, but you didn't" to "You agreed not to fuck Laura, then you fucked Laura." It's beneficial to the relationship, and keeps the drama to a minimum, if your response is appropriate to what agreement was violated. Overreacting only adds fuel to the fire.

The first step toward resolution is for everyone involved to acknowledge what happened and talk about it. Begin by giving yourself and your partner the benefit of the doubt: no one is perfect; we all make mistakes. Next, think about the circumstances: was this a case of miscommunication, a gray area, bad timing, or a total disregard of the rules? Thus begins the process of digging to see why the violation occurred: what were the person's intentions, what were the motivating factors? Sometimes people break rules in the heat of the moment, when they're just not thinking clearly. The instance could be circumstantial and simply a case of bad judgment. Or the behavior may signal something deeper. Did the person who broke the rule act out of anger, resentment, jealousy, or revenge?

Sometimes people think a rule is unfairly restrictive, agree to it anyway, then go on to break it. Not adhering to an agreement can be a passive-aggressive way to get a partner's attention or retaliate for a previous incident. Some people simply don't like rules; they often test an agreed-to boundary to see what they can get away with, how far they can push it. If a pattern develops where someone is constantly breaking the rules, you should ask yourself whether that person is trustworthy.

Among the people I interviewed, blatant and deliberate agreement violations were considered the most serious. Interestingly, the most common of these were equivalent to cheating:

- A partner has unprotected or unsafe sex with someone they're not fluid-bonded with.
- Someone sees a partner they agreed not to see (whether temporarily or permanently).
- A partner has sex with someone without prior permission.
- Someone begins a new relationship without checking in with existing partners.

Ingrid recounts what happened when her husband broke one of their rules:

> Shortly after my husband and I talked about opening up our relationship, he slept with my best friend, Adrienne. I suppose she is our best friend, but nevertheless, he did not have previous permission, which [was] a violation of the rules we'd set up, and therefore cheating. After a lot of soul-searching and some arguments, I came to the conclusion that if he had to break the rules or make a mistake, this was probably the "best of the worst," so to speak. We both love Adrienne, and we'd been involved with her sexually before in a threesome, so it wasn't a far stretch. She did know of our relationship status and thought he had prior permission, and he admitted his mistake to both Adrienne and myself right away the next morning. We revised the rules to clearly state that permission must be explicitly given beforehand, and we're working through it.

Sandra is a member of a five-person polyamorous circle in which all members are faithful within the group. "My husband had an affair with the next-door neighbor, which was incredibly convenient for him, and bad timing. Everybody was a little pissed off about it. He didn't bother asking for permission or even telling anybody for about three months, which is just bad form. He told us from the other side of the planet [he was out of the country]. I was really pissed off, because, you know, you don't *do that*."

In another instance, one member of the circle wanted to have a relationship with a friend of the family:

> *She mentioned to three of us that she was interested in this friend, but not to our girlfriend on the East Coast. She said, "I'm interested in pursuing this sort-of relationship with this person." And I said, "That's interesting, let me know how that develops," because the rules are you ask for permission and get permission before you initiate intimacy. She didn't bother doing that. She thought that just mentioning it was tacit approval. Well, I don't know if she actually thought that or she was just trying to get away with it, but at any rate I found out about it in an unpleasant way. After being intimate with this friend of the family, she was intimate with her husband, who is my partner. He told my girlfriend, and she turned around to me and said, "Gee, I can't believe you're being so casual about this thing that happened." And I said, "What?" I hadn't heard of it, so I was furious. I was really angry. It was almost a deal breaker.*

As these examples show, open relationships are not immune from cheating. Resolving problems like these takes patience, time, and understanding. The person who made the mistake has to take responsibility for their behavior and apologize. When someone breaks a rule, people feel confused, hurt, and betrayed—those feelings do not heal overnight. Trust must be reestablished between partners, and that takes time. The broken rule may signal that one of your agreements needs to change; perhaps one partner wants an amendment to accommodate some new desire or person. You may find that you need to renegotiate your terms so that they reflect a shift in the relationship. Agreements should be dynamic, just like the people and relationships behind them.

Seeking Help

There are books, websites, and workshops on open relationships that can be of great help when facing problems. When dealing with common issues, it is useful to talk to other people in open relationships. Whether it's through an online community or a Listserv or, even better, a face-to-face support group, reach out to people who have experience to share. Peer-based support and advice from knowledgeable folks who've grappled with similar issues can be invaluable. (See the Resource Guide for more information.)

Individuals, couples, and polyfidelitous groups who face challenges in their nonmonogamous relationships can also benefit from some form of counseling. An objective, experienced, compassionate therapist can help you to explore the underlying issues in your conflicts, communicate and understand one another's perspectives better, and resolve problems.

Unfortunately, many professionals in psychology and psychiatry (and other medical fields) still have little education or experience when it comes to ethical, responsible nonmonogamy. Mainstream textbooks and courses in relationships and family structures rarely include information about nonmonogamy and polyamory.[5] Some professionals believe that any form of nonmonogamy—even when consensual—is dysfunctional and pathological. Nonmonogamy is not by its nature a psychological problem. Nonmonogamous people deserve mental health care from open-minded, knowledgeable professionals.

Whether you seek a psychoanalyst, a therapist, or a relationship coach, it's important for you to find a professional who believes non-monogamy is a valid choice and who has experience in counseling nonmonogamous clients. It is not your responsibility to spend time educating a therapist about nonmonogamy or arguing with him about its validity. For some resources on finding a professional, see the Resource Guide at the end of the book.

IN HER OWN WORDS: DANI

"An alternative style of marriage has made my marriage stronger."

DANI, 32, lives in Illinois, where she is an ordained minister serving in a mainline Christian denomination. She has been married to her husband for 13 years, but they no longer have a sexual relationship. He has little interest in sex. When she discovered her bisexuality and her desire for BDSM, everything changed in her life. Today, her marriage is open; she considers her husband her primary partner, her Master her other primary partner, and she has several nonprimary relationships. Her husband dates other women, but does not have sex with them.

"[When I came out about being bi and kinky] I said, I love you, I still want to be married to you, but if I don't have sex, one of us is going to die, and it's not going to be me. We fought about it, we talked about divorce, and it was nasty. Finally he said, 'Well, I just don't want to know. I don't want to know much, I don't want to know details. You can tell me who, you can tell me when, but I don't want to know anything else.'... It changed everything. We stopped fighting at home, because we weren't fighting about sex anymore... We'd been married for 10 years and at that point it had been a topic for us for, like, six.

I truly believe that being in an alternative style of marriage has made my marriage stronger because now we can focus on the things that make us a good couple. My husband and I have a lot of things in common... We love to read the same kinds of books, skiing, movies, and outdoor adventure sports. We love to do these things together... The two major issues that my husband [and I] would fight over besides money—and everybody fights over money, that's just life—were religion and sex. Taking those out of the picture and getting those two needs filled elsewhere has given us the opportunity to build on all of the other really good stuff that we have, so we're just a stronger couple. I can't even imagine divorcing him now. He drives me crazy and sometimes I want to strangle him, but divorce him, no. Because I love him very much. And we can focus on our strengths as a couple so much more now. He's not checking off the list of his needs that are not getting met, and I'm not checking off the list of my needs that are not getting met, because they're getting met by other relationships.

Finding a Master who can fulfill my faith and BDSM needs as well as my sexual needs has made me a more complete, more healthy person. I couldn't be luckier to have such wonderful people in my life… [My husband] is very giving and he likes to see me happy. My happiness is what's important to him, and his happiness is important to me. So for this to make me happy and to make our marriage better really worked out great for us."

Chapter 15

Opening Up Again:
When Something Changes

CHANGE IS DIFFICULT in all relationships, but it can occur frequently in open relationships. New experiences, sexual partners, and relationship partners come in and out of your lives; they shake up existing relationship dynamics, influence feelings, shift commitments, and wreak havoc if you're not equipped to deal with them. What follows are some of the more significant changes commonly experienced by nonmonogamous people, along with some strategies for coping with them.

> We tend to think of relationships as static, as if we could just get into them, assume a position inside them and then continue to hold it, essentially without changing forever, world without end. But in fact, our relationships are fluid, vivid, mercurial, and constantly changing.
> —DAPHNE ROSE KINGMA[1]

A New Desire

When one partner discovers she has a new desire—for a partner of a different gender, a new sexual activity, or BDSM, for example—it can come as a surprise to her other partners. If you are the partner with the new desire, it's your responsibility to share it, allow your partner(s) some time and space to process the new information, and be available to discuss their questions or concerns. This is a good time to reassure them that though this new thing will change your relationship, it doesn't diminish it. Invite your partner(s) to take part in exploring it, if that's possible, but also allow them the freedom to decline to participate. If your partner doesn't share your newfound desire, don't be dismayed. Let go of the myth that you will be 100 percent sexually compatible with a partner—it's not a requirement, it's not reasonable, and it is rare.

If your partner has informed you about a new desire of his, it's common to feel shocked, overwhelmed, confused, and threatened. Don't let your own insecurities get the best of you in these situations; fight hard to see the change for what it is and not as a comment on you, the relationship, or the shortcomings of either. Sometimes, you believe you know your partner so well that a radical change catches you off guard and you suddenly question your connection. This is the "I thought I knew you" reaction; remember that you *do* know your partner, and now he is inviting you to know even more of him. Rather than focus on the negative ("How long have you been wanting this and not telling me?"), try to focus on the positive: he has given you a gift based on how much he trusts and values you in his life.

A New Orientation

Probably one of the most dramatic announcements of a new desire can come when one spouse in a heterosexual marriage comes out as gay or lesbian. Couples who decide to open up their relationship as a result face the added pressure of grappling with the change in sexual orientation. Because the spouse who comes out is having a life-changing experience, Amity Buxton cautions spouses to anticipate this element of the transition:

> Be prepared for a good period of disorientation; as the gay/bi spouse discovers the other side, the excitement of the

discoveries [may] blind the spouse for a while to the positives of the heterosexual relationship. If the straight spouse can hold it together and remain open and love at this crucial time, when the gay/bi partner calms down, the marriage will be better than ever.[2]

In addition to coping with one spouse's euphoria over coming out, both partners in mixed-orientation marriages must let go of the fairy tale of the perfect white-picket-fence marriage, and they have to grieve that loss. They must figure out what each person needs to stay in the relationship and be fulfilled. They have to confront issues of homophobia—their own and others'. Some carry the burden of maintaining appearances, keeping their secret from loved ones; others tell friends and family, and must deal with criticism, ignorance, and rejection.

While it is important for mixed-orientation couples to have the support of loved ones, it's often more helpful to seek support from people who have been in a similar situation. Finding a group (whether online or in person) as well as an experienced therapist can help you navigate the unfamiliar waters.

A New Relationship

The inability to know what the future holds when someone you love very deeply is starting a new relationship is hard to deal with. [The new relationship] hasn't had enough time to develop to know what kind of impact it might have on your own. —Lena

When you are in one or more relationships and someone new enters the picture, things inevitably change. If you are interested in a new partner, first follow the rules you have agreed to, whether it's asking permission before getting involved, keeping people in the loop, or setting up a face-to-face meeting between existing partners and the newbie. Whatever it is you said you'd do—do it. People are much more likely to respond positively when they feel that you've been aboveboard with them. "I had unsafe sex with this guy and now I want to start a relationship with him" is a poor way to introduce the person. Even though NRE has started to kick in, pace yourself. Don't rush into spending every weekend together or get matching tattoos. Let yourself—and your existing partner(s)—get used to the idea.

If your partner has begun a new relationship, feel free to renegotiate limits, time, and other matters now that there is an additional partner in her life. Make sure she is spending enough time with you so you don't feel neglected. Remind yourself that this new relationship is not about you. Tell the voice in your head shouting *She wants this change, so it must mean she's not happy with me!* to buzz off. If you're feeling insecure, reach out to other loved ones for support. Ask your partner for reassurance. Remember, she's drunk on NRE, so be prepared to be frustrated or annoyed with her.

Ginger is a 33-year-old human resources director from Baltimore; she has been married to her husband, Craig, for five years, and they practice BDSM. During the first four years of their marriage, the two of them played with other women only. About a year ago, they met a woman named Tonya and began playing with her; subsequently, they discussed the possibility of including Tonya's husband, Nat. One night, the three were doing a scene and invited Nat to watch. After the threesome played for a while, Craig (as Ginger's Dominant) directed Ginger to go off by herself and have sex with Nat. Ginger was surprised, but also excited, because she was attracted to Nat. Ginger and Nat really clicked that night and continued to see each other. She expressed to her husband that she had developed deep feelings for Nat, and Craig freaked out. Ginger says:

> I didn't realize that Craig hadn't seen it coming. I was, like, "Oh, isn't this great?" and he was having full-out panic attacks, shortness of breath, hyperventilating, crying. I've hardly ever seen this

guy cry. At that point, we'd been seeing Nat and Tonya for a couple of months and I was really bonded with Nat—and with Tonya. Craig wanted to call off the whole relationship. I'd say, "Okay we won't see them anymore," but then I was mad. The more upset Craig got, the more jealous and possessive he became. Nat and I made plans to meet secretly. When Craig found out about it, there was an explosion, and that's when we stopped seeing them completely.

Ginger and Craig continued to fight about it. "In his heart of hearts, Craig felt that we started out being poly with women only, and gosh darn it, that's the way we should stay." They had different visions of their polyamory, and their visions didn't mesh. Ginger considered leaving Craig:

It wasn't that I didn't love him. It was that he wanted to keep me in this box that I didn't want to be in. He saw that we agreed from the beginning about having other women in our relationship and that I was breaking our agreement. I see things a lot more fluid and gray and he sees things as more black and white... He never envisioned poly involving other men, at least not men I'd fall in love with. He was feeling unloved, unworthy, disposable, jealous, not in control, hurt. Unfortunately, I was already in love with Nat by this time, and couldn't give him up without breaking my heart. After learning to be poly and share my husband with other women, and living that life for over four years, I felt entitled to explore my feelings for Nat... I didn't see a solution, because I didn't think he would ever agree to see Tonya and Nat anymore, and I didn't think I'd be happy not seeing them.

Ginger and Craig went to couples counseling, where Craig worked on his anger and insecurity. One day, Craig arranged for the four of them to have dinner. Ginger says, "I don't know if it was counseling, I don't know if was the fear of losing our relationship," but Craig announced at dinner he wanted to reconcile. A few weeks later, Nat and Ginger began to have a regular weekly date night. Craig was finally willing to accept him in Ginger's life, with one caveat: Ginger would not have any other male partners. So, they renegotiated their agreement to reflect these new terms.

Falling in Love

Ginger acknowledges that another reason her relationship with Nat was difficult for her husband to deal with was that she had such strong feelings for Nat. Many people in open relationships struggle when love becomes part of the equation. Some people's agreements allow for the possibility of deep emotional relationships—even love— with other partners. But this doesn't make it any easier when your partner announces she's fallen in love with someone else. One reason it stirs up such strong emotions is the myth of monogamy: we are taught that you can only be in love with one person at a time. In the monogamous world, a partner's declaration of love for someone else usually means the present relationship is over.

In nonmonogamy, a new love does not mean the loss of the relationship, but it may still feel like a loss: loss of security, loss of time, loss of affection, or loss of status (as the only primary, as the only one he loves, and so on). A statement of love for someone new can intensify uncertainty: when she was a casual partner, you felt secure, but now that he *loves* her… Embracing your partner's love for someone new is part of achieving compersion. To get there, you must try to feel not loss, but gain: your partner has gained a new love, which brings more love into your world.

One of the more difficult issues Khane had to deal with was hearing his primary partner, Ignacio, express his love for some of his other partners. "I had a lot of residual issues from my past relationship. I felt that we would stray away from being primaries and I didn't want that to happen. I prepared for the worst," Khane says. Ignacio wanted to reassure Khane, but also be realistic: "I couldn't really say, 'Well, that'll never happen, baby,' because it's not true; it could happen... Right now I love the hell out of him. I can't even think of having another primary. I could say, 'Right now, in this moment, I don't want that.'" Processing and renegotiating this issue brought up difficult questions for Khane:

> I was able to ask myself honest questions like, What if I had announced my love for another person first? What would be different right now—am I being fair? What are my fears, and what is needed to quell them? What really makes our relationship primary? Am I suffering from leftover monogamous thoughts? Am I really polyamorous? I came to realize that like all the other times we've gone through rough moments, it was just another growing point, [a] chance to see if we could actually walk the [walk]... It's easy to have a primary and be polyamorous when neither person feels love for another partner.

Khane and Ignacio's experience demonstrates some important points. They take promises seriously. When they reassure one another, they talk about what's happening in the present rather than make a guarantee of forever. They embrace uncertainty. They are committed to "walking the walk" of polyamory: calling yourself poly means accepting the reality of falling in love with other people.

But what if falling in love was not part of your agreement? That's a different ball of wax. Let's say you practice a style of nonmonogamy where loving more than one partner is not part of your agreement. You've abided by the rules and had only casual sex partners outside the relationship, but one day find yourself experiencing more intense feelings for one of them. First, you must come clean to your partner. Then begins the harder work: what will you do about it? Some people who have this experience break off the relationship with the new partner to preserve the primary partnership. Others renegotiate the terms of their relationship to accommodate additional loving relationships. What you do depends on what you and your partner want and the needs of the primary relationship.

From Monogamous to Nonmonogamous

If you are in a monogamous relationship and are considering some style of nonmonogamy, chances are both partners did not raise the issue simultaneously—one of you approached the other about it. If you initiated the conversation, make sure to give your partner plenty of time and space to think it over. Point him to books, websites, and other resources, and then let him absorb the information at his own pace. If your partner was the one who brought it up, do not feel pressured to make a decision right away. Do your research, give it careful consideration, ask questions, and be sure before you decide.

If you decide to try nonmonogamy, the transition can be a rocky one. When a couple moves from monogamy to nonmonogamy, cracks in the relationship are often exposed and magnified. Therapist Joy Davidson says: "When primary partners bring up the issue of nonmonogamy for the first time: a) the relationship paradigm is immediately altered; b) [the] conversation forces the exploration of needs that are not being met and emotional secrets that have been kept."[3] Confronting the dysfunctional patterns, unmet needs, and other demons in your relationship is not easy, and this could be a good time to seek counseling. You want to resolve any major conflicts and issues and bring the relationship to a place of stability *before* you explore nonmonogamy. If you don't, things are likely to go awry very quickly. As you think about what style of nonmonogamy you'd like to try, be honest about what you want.

When you begin actually being nonmonogamous, the dynamics between you and your partner will likely change. It's very difficult, but necessary, to let go of your monogamous baggage and any investment

> ### Reflecting on Change
>
> Coping with change is an important skill to learn. Once you get over the shock and disorientation it inevitably brings, ask yourself these questions:
>
> - How does this change affect my current relationship(s)?
> - What are the negative implications of this change?
> - What scares me about this change?
> - What are the positive implications of this change?
> - What pleases me about this change?
> - What do I need to help make the transition brought on by this change easier?

you had in "the way things used to be." For example, in the beginning of his relationship with Lucy, Theo believed that Lucy avoided telling him when she wanted to hook up with other people because it brought up old upsets:

> When she was in Boston and I was in New York, she would call and say, "I'm on my way home. I'll call you when I get home, and we'll have our nightly check-in." Then she would disappear and end up screwing somebody... She didn't want to deal with talking to me about it. She was turned on and wanted to go play, and she didn't want to have to hash it out... When people are not experienced in nonmonogamy, talking about being with somebody else has the emotional charge of all this history: whether you cheated on somebody or whether you were dating more than one person, having to deal with [other people's] upsets—all that stuff people don't want to confront.

Theo's observation shows how you can unconsciously revert to the restrictive ideas of monogamy. If you played by all the unspoken rules of monogamy when you were in your monogamous relationship, you learned some things you're going to have to unlearn: That you should feel love and sexual desire only for your partner. That you must not tell your spouse you find another person attractive, you've developed a crush, you like flirting with someone, you want to have sex with them, or you have a fantasy about them. That one person can fulfill all your needs; if you have a need your partner cannot or does not want to meet, file it away, because you're out of luck. Accepting that you can be attracted to, have sex with, and love more than one person can be hard. Learning to talk about wants and needs that involve people other than your partner is not something we are taught. Communicating in a totally new way will take some time and getting used to.

When you first adopt nonmonogamy, go slowly. Ruth and her partner began fantasizing about what it would be like to have a third partner, and they swapped stories before they actually did anything. Ruth believes this helped them grow comfortable with the idea and distill what was important to them. Now she and her partner are part of a triad.

When George and Emma first decided to open up their relationship, George says:

> At first, for a while, we did the team thing. [We said] we can be involved with somebody else, but it has to be both of us. Then we started branching out to the idea of having experiences separately, and we both had those. We had a lot of the jealousy issues along the way, a lot of 'I'm not getting attention paid to me' and 'You're out [while] I'm stuck at home.' There was a little bit of on and off: let's not be open, quite so open, how are we going to structure this, how are we going to do this. We went back and forth figuring out how we actually wanted to do this poly thing.

They eventually became part of a closed triad with Penny. Recently, the three decided to open up the triad, and this change has been another challenge:

> It's at a time when none of us has somebody immediately. A lot of times, opening up happens because 'Oh my god, there's this person I'm interested in, here's this opportunity, let's open up so I can take advantage of this opportunity!' That skews things rather badly. Drawing on our past problems and mistakes, [we said] we were interested in having this kind of relationship, so why don't we go ahead and proactively take this step before anybody is in the position of being forced to or having to advocate for it—before there's any other weird dynamic layered on top of it.

George believes they made the transition from closed to open smoothly due to the fact that there was no one waiting in the wings.

You may be single with a history of monogamous relationships when you decide to become nonmonogamous. When Madeline, a 35-year-old mother and massage therapist from the Midwest, ended her marriage, she decided to become nonmonogamous:

> It was a conscious decision... It was six or eight months after we separated before I was interested in dating anybody or going out or even having sex with anybody... I started going out with this guy, we hit it off, and it was very clear from the beginning that this was not going to be serious. Neither one of us was interested in having a boyfriend or a girlfriend... Very gradually, other casual things started happening... I thought to myself, this is what my life was like in college or in my early 20s, where I don't have to be tied down to one person. In fact, it's rather nice to have this choice of different people who will fulfill different needs. I think the decision wasn't necessarily conscious but it became this revelation that, yeah, I can do this and this is good for me. I never [do]

anything behind anyone's back. I don't tell everyone everything,
but everyone I'm seeing knows that I see other people.

Samiya is a 36-year-old bisexual African American woman who
works in government and lives in Maryland. After ending an eight-year
lesbian relationship, she thought her dissatisfaction was with the specific
relationship. But then she began seeing someone new and questioned if
monogamy was right for her:

> *A few years ago I was dating another bi woman. She liked to play*
> *around quite a bit and experiment. At that time, I came to real-*
> *ize that there were certain things I want that I would never have*
> *in that relationship… I just knew that if I were with her indefinitely*
> *I would still want to seek out [other experiences], not because I*
> *didn't love her but because that's what I need to feel balance.*

When she embraced nonmonogamy, it changed other aspects of her
life:

> *I started really asking myself: What is it that I want? What is it*
> *that I need? And spending some time just with myself, not going*
> *according to what other people said I should be, that's when*
> *things developed more freely… The funny thing about living this*
> *truth about myself is that I feel able to live the truth in other*
> *areas of my life… Once I was able to admit this for myself and*
> *live it, I don't have the desire to run around hiding things. I don't*
> *try to be so-called nice about my ideas or my views in other*
> *areas—whether it's work, friendship, family.*

Making the transition from monogamy to nonmonogamy requires
patience. Give yourself time to reframe how you think about and share
your desire for other people. Go slowly, pace yourself—don't jump
into having a secondary partner, two fuck buddies, and a lover all in
one month. Make agreements with your partners and stick to them.

From Nonmonogamous to Monogamous

This book has dealt nearly entirely with nonmonogamy, but there are plenty of instances when nonmonogamous relationships become monogamous. Sometimes the change is temporary. When the people I interviewed talked about shifting from nonmonogamy to monogamy for a fixed period of time, it usually came about as a way of addressing a problem, reconnecting and reestablishing trust, or coping with some significant change or crisis. For example, Leslie and her triad partners Ed and Colin decided to close their triad to additional partners while Leslie received treatment for cancer. Barbara's partner chose a period of monogamy for himself to deal with an addiction. When my partner moved across the country to live with me, we decided to be monogamous for six months while he settled into a new city, a new job, basically a whole new life. With so much for him to adjust to, I wanted to give him a sense of security and let him know that he would be my priority.

Gabrielle, a 32-year-old Native American woman from Seattle, has had mostly polyamorous relationships; in fact, only two of her 20 relationships have been monogamous. Her current primary relationship with her husband, Jeff, started as polyamorous five and a half years ago. Recently, a woman began pursuing Jeff:

> She had been playing with a lot of friends of ours. As soon as she would get involved with a man and have sex with him, she would basically just dump him like a hot potato. She was going through most of our friends and doing that. When she was pursuing them, she was really dominating their time and treating their partners like crap. She started doing this with me, and I said, "No, I'm not comfortable with this chick, she's really freaking me out, and she really pisses me off."

Gabrielle vetoed the woman, but Jeff played with her anyway. Gabrielle felt betrayed. She asked him to be monogamous with her so they could work on reestablishing their trust. She became monogamous as well:

I just wanted to decomplicate the relationship. I thought if I was going to ask him to be monogamous with me, I needed to make the same commitment to him; that was pretty much just an equality and fairness thing. I didn't think he was being malicious with what happened. I just thought we needed some time rebuilding our relationship, rebuilding our trust... It was hard to give up my relationships... [especially] the guy I was pretty serious about. I still miss him. But it was necessary so that my primary relationship could move forward.

The tight-knit poly community to which Gabrielle and her husband belonged began to ostracize them:

As soon as we decided to be monogamous, within a matter of weeks we stopped getting invited to parties, stopped getting invited to our friends' houses, and all of our poly friends stopped having time to spend with us... It seems that if you're not poly, then it threatens their existence. They're very insecure about being poly and want only people who are like them or accept them to be around them.

The lack of support has been very difficult, but Gabrielle believes monogamy is what she and her husband need right now. They are open to exploring nonmonogamy again once they have worked on their issues.

Some people decide to try monogamy and agree to it for the fore-seeable future. Nonmonogamous people who strongly believe in open relationships and make them a philosophical preference can become deeply invested in them. If you've spent a lot of thought and energy rejecting traditional monogamy, it may seem as if you're stepping back-ward to decide your relationship should be monogamous. If you are considering this option, know that it doesn't mean you have failed at nonmonogamy or that you're buying into society's norms.

People's self-judgment can be exacerbated by criticism from other nonmonogamous people. Some polyamorous people believe so strongly in polyamory as a lifestyle that they see other styles—even other styles of nonmonogamy—as inferior. Some people see polyamory as an orientation, like sexual orientation, and believe that there is no equivalent to bisexuality: you're either nonmonogamous or you're not. People can become catty and mean when defending their community, as happened with Gabrielle when she first met other poly people and asked them about their lifestyle: "Everyone was like, 'Oh, it's so wonderful' and 'It's all about not owning your partner.' They made it sound like this superior lifestyle, this superior way of thinking and being, as if you'd be a better person for doing it. [They said that] monogamous people are really just enslaved to each other."

If you've explored your options and chosen monogamy, remember that your choice is valid. You seek a relationship style that fits your needs, and for some people that style is monogamy. Take all the relationship skills you learned from nonmonogamy and apply them to your monogamous relationship.

From Primary to Nonprimary

In the world of monogamy, there are usually two choices when something isn't working: stay together or break up. For polyamorous people, there are many more options; for instance, the relationship can continue—only in a different form. When a primary relationship becomes nonprimary, it still feels like a kind of breakup. You must grieve the loss, but also take comfort in the fact that the relationship can evolve into something else that works for both partners.

When Lena and Sal met, they had a common interest in community activism and worked on forming a local poly organization together.

They formed a strong bond, moved in together, and became primary partners for nearly eight years. Both had other relationship partners during that time. Lena describes how their relationship changed:

> There were some serious things that were not really available in my relationship with Sal. We're actually very different in a lot of ways. He's a lovely man and I love him to death, but there were some fairly significant compatibility issues for living together. I was pacing myself because I'd been on the poly roller coaster earlier in my poly years and I was done with having a lot of drama, so I wasn't out actively searching for new partners. But then I met Gavin and we clicked so beautifully, our values were so much the same… About the same time, Sal met Jennie. I liked Jennie a lot and she liked me, and we all spent some time together, but it was pretty clear that Sal and Jennie were more compatible than he and I were. It was this serendipity thing that happened: I fell madly in love with Gavin, Sal fell in love with Jennie. We had a heart-to-heart talk [where we discussed] that these were serious relationships and they felt like a better fit. One of the beautiful parts of polyamory to me is that you don't have to ditch the whole relationship; you can change it to be something more suitable to what you want, what your needs are, what everybody's needs are.

After Lena began spending more time with Gavin and Sal began spending more time with Jennie, everyone sat down and talked about logistics: who lived where, when leases would expire, financial issues. They devised a plan to shift living arrangements so Lena and Gavin would move in together and Sal would move in with another partner of his. Lena credits the fairly smooth transition to their dedication to one another and their pride in being leaders in their poly community:

> The key was that Sal and I loved each other and wanted to be happy. We had over time agreed that we didn't intend to own each

other, even if it meant giving each other up to someone else because it made us happier. We agreed that it would be painful too, [but] we wanted to have enough love in our hearts to be able to do that... I long ago gave up the notion of "till death do us part." What made the difference for Sal and me was that we both have enough pride in being people who represent polyamory that we don't want to be the ones in the big stink.

The transition from primary to nonprimary can be difficult just in terms of logistics, especially if you live together, share finances, jointly own property, or co-parent children. In these difficult moments, put to use what you've learned through the practice of polyamory: self-reflection, honesty, communication, boundaries. If necessary, ask a therapist or relationship coach to help you with the transition.

Coping with Change

Acknowledge and embrace the change that comes with your open relationship. Expect it, so that it doesn't sneak up on you and catch you completely off guard. Change disrupts, threatens the status quo, and makes us feel insecure. If you perceive change as a negative force, it can overwhelm, intimidate, and paralyze you. However, if you see change as something positive—an opportunity to learn and grow—it can feel like a gift. Change in someone else can be just as surprising as change in yourself. When you experience change in yourself, you know that it will affect you. But when a partner comes to you and announces that something is changing or has changed, it may affect you in unexpected ways. It's the domino effect: their change means that we must change.

Change inspires a range of emotions, and people's reactions to change can differ greatly. It can produce confusion: "When I met you, you weren't into BDSM; now all of a sudden you are?" It can feel like a form of betrayal: "But this is what we agreed to, this is what I signed up for; now you're changing the rules." Change can hit the core of someone's deepest insecurities: "You want this change, so it must mean you're not happy *with me*." It can also make people angry: "We agreed to partnered nonmonogamy; now you tell me you want to be polyamorous?" At the heart of many negative reactions to change is fear: fear of the unknown, fear of things being different, fear of the relationship ending. You've got to face the fear head on, otherwise it can swallow you whole.

Change is an opportunity to sit down with your partner(s) and evaluate your relationship. Examine your rules and agreements thus far and see what needs to be amended to accommodate the change. Begin the negotiation process again: consider where you are, who you are, what you need and want. You may want to start fresh, with a blank sheet of paper; let all past agreements go and begin again. The goals are the same as when you first negotiated your agreement: listen to each other, ask for what you want, and be willing to compromise.

While change does not have to signal the end of a relationship, sometimes a change can be so profound that the relationship cannot continue. If accommodating the change means you must unduly compromise your most basic needs and wants, it may be time to move on. Some changes are relationship deal breakers. When Jimmy, a 42-year-old transgendered man from Pittsburgh, began a new primary relationship, two of his other relationships ended:

> *I had two longtime loves that contributed a great deal to my life. The relationships were rich with love, sex, and learning. When I fell in love with my current partner, it felt to them like a violation of our relationship. At that time I was poly/nonpartnering. Neither of them was primary and they believed there never would be someone primary. It was a big change in the way I was living my life to be enthralled with a love in a way I might want to live*

with her. I did not manage their concerns well. I asserted my right to grow as I needed and that the change was not breaking a promise. Ultimately, I find it harder to grow and change dynamically in a half-dozen committed relationships than in one. But, the trade-off of greater complexity in exchange for diverse connection remains worth it.

Ending a relationship is difficult, disruptive, and painful. Breakups can bring out the worst in many people. We have few models for a clean, loving, and graceful end to a relationship. But, as clichéd as it may sound, breaking up can be yet another opportunity for growth: you can let go of old patterns, learn from past mistakes, achieve clarity about what you want, and move forward with your life.

PROFILE: ANDI AND JOSH

"We're not as naïve as we were."

ANDI, AN EVENT PLANNER, AND JOSH, a construction manager, both 30, live in New York City and have been together for eight years. They met in college, where they dated for several years, and in 1999 they were married. Andi was a virgin until their wedding night, and their premarital relationship had been monogamous. After four years of monogamous marriage, Andi expressed interest in women, and Josh told her he was open to her exploring her bisexuality. Around that time, they hooked up with a male friend of theirs for their first threesome; it was a positive experience for both of them. Then Andi began dating and having sex with women. Since Josh had revealed that he, too, might be bisexual, Andi told him it was all right with her if he dated men.

Josh was more interested in doing things together, so they put an ad on a website and eventually met and had sex with another couple.

They also began having sex with others on their own, adopting a style of partnered nonmonogamy: "At that point, the fact of the matter was we had our primary relationship and everything else was just sexual fun things," Josh says. After reading *The Ethical Slut*, they talked about other possibilities and fantasized about finding another bi couple to have a relationship with. They dabbled in dating others—Andi dated men and women, and Josh dated women. They opened the door to the possibility of falling in love. "He had been dating this girl for a while. I would say it was the most emotional relationship I ever saw [him] have outside our relationship," Andi says. "I remember asking him, 'Do you think you're falling in love with her?' I think he said, 'I'm not sure.' I said, 'Well, I'm okay with that, you know. Love is a great feeling.'"

Wanting to invest more emotional energy in their other partners, they started seeking girlfriends and boyfriends rather than just casual sex partners. At that point, they had a full disclosure rule, Josh says. "Basically, I called it 'Don't ask, do tell.' We didn't want to be surprised by anything. We wanted to be proactive and forthcoming."

For Andi, polyamory worked on several levels: "It's really good to get attention from other people to increase our confidence. For me, it gave me a lot of experience I never had. Growing up Catholic, with Josh my first lover, and never having been with other women, I felt I was deprived of sexual experiences and emotional relationships. [I had the chance to] build those emotional relationships with men and women, get to know people, and make deep connections. Then we also had this idea that [polyamory] made our relationship stronger because: a) we're being so open and honest with each other; and b) you need a really secure relationship to go outside of it. We felt very proud of ourselves that we have that and always try to maintain that—it made that bond even stronger."

"Along with the confidence came a growing and improving sex life," Josh says. They brought what they learned from other relationships back to their partnership. They also took good care of themselves, worked out, and cared more about how they looked while they were dating other people.

Josh and Andi struggled with jealousy over the amount of time each spent with other partners. "Balance was the big [conflict]... It was very difficult when one of us had a relationship going on outside, especially something serious, and one of us didn't," Andi says. "Or if I was dating a lot, because it was a lot easier for a married woman to get dates—with men or women." Josh agrees: "If Andi's dating three guys and I've got nothing going on the side for myself, it was very difficult." But they managed their jealousy, they fell in love with other people, and they had several relationships.

About a year ago, Josh began seeing a new woman. Andi says, "This got really serious. It was the first time I was afraid of it affecting our relationship." Josh says, "I know I did some things that were neglectful, like breaking plans with my wife to hang out with this other girl." While Andi was trying hard to accept this new partner, one night when she and Josh met for drinks Josh started making out with *another* woman, a former student of his from his teaching years. It was too much for Andi, and they had a horrific argument.

After the fight, they agreed to take a month apart and Andi moved out—just weeks before their seventh wedding anniversary. "I still knew that we belonged together. I had this epiphany: We have to give up all this other stuff, we have to go to couples therapy," Andi says. "We had to really focus on each other. For the first time in three and a half or four years, I said I could be monogamous again." That was a big revelation for her. "Once we were poly, I identified so much with it, it made me happy, I felt fulfilled, I felt so much more like myself... It was really, really important to me. [There were previous times when] he wanted to go back to being monogamous, and I said I couldn't do it."

This time was different, Andi says. "I thought, this all makes so much more sense now, we've totally been neglecting each other, our needs aren't getting met. I think we've been putting on a front. We would be jealous and say, Oh, it's okay, we'll just work through it. We'd have real paralyzing fears sometimes. Something bad would happen, but we'd say it's going to be fine. Legitimate, deep, awful feelings that we were having—we blew them off as just part of the relationship, stuff that will just make us stronger. Finally I [said] we had to address all these issues, and do it in couples therapy, because we were so distant from each other at that point."

While Josh had pressed for monogamy in the past, now that Andi was ready to try it Josh didn't want to. He was in love with his new partner and didn't want to stop seeing her. Andi ended her other relationships, but Josh resisted. Andi says, "Even though I was committed at that point that we had to be monogamous, I thought, What can I do? I have to accept this, basically. Eventually he'll figure it out and we'll be together. I did not think it was going to last with them anyway. Then Josh came to the realization on his own that he had to put a hundred and ten percent into our relationship if there was ever a chance that it would survive. We had to put everything we had into it. It was the only way we would know if we had a real shot."

They went into couples counseling and worked on communicating better. They don't believe that polyamory was the cause of their near breakup. Josh says, "[polyamory] would exacerbate small problems and magnify, amplify everything… I felt that it may have brought things to the surface that we were struggling with anyway—communication issues that may have dragged on for years and years that maybe would never have erupted. But with all the additional stresses on our relationship because of the polyamory, everything came to a head and we had no choice but to deal with it."

After a year of monogamy and couples counseling, they recently celebrated their eighth wedding anniversary. They have worked hard to repair their relationship, and they feel confident and connected. While they haven't sworn off polyamory for good, they are cautious about it. Andi says, "We've made out with other people. We haven't dated anybody else, and I don't know if we'll go down that road. I think it's a lot more scary to us now. We're not as naïve as we were… I'd still like to have other experiences, but it's complicated. It does put a stress on our relationship and it's not always safe, and those are big factors… I'm still okay with having some sexual experiences with other people, especially if we're doing it together. I think it could be really fun. Relationships—not so much. I think that's where a lot of the problems came from: we were totally distracted by our emotions for these other people." "I'm a bit more nervous about it all," Josh says. "A little bit of making out here and there is fairly harmless. But outside sexual relationships when we're not together feels threatening to me. It just brings back a lot of the memories—positive memories, but also of all the things that went wrong."

"It was very much a learning experience," Andi says. "Figuring out that I'm bisexual was a huge thing for me… I think I realized, as we started to be more picky and more safe, I was trying to figure out what I was looking for. I really wanted the deep emotional relationships, which was something I felt I didn't really have a lot of before Josh. I think I was seeking deeper relationships through our polyamory. All our closest friends right now we've probably had some sort of sexual relationship with at some point. Our friends have changed over the years, and I feel we have deeper, more meaningful relationships, more open relationships, with the people we're friends with now. We're just more open people in general, and I like that. I think it's more *us*."

Chapter 16

Coming Out (or Not), Finding Community, Creating Families

HAVING READ THIS FAR, you've learned some skills for creating the open relationship that's right for you and your partner(s). Now it's time to deal with the world at large. In this chapter, we'll explore some of the different ways you relate to the people around you: coming out about your nonmonogamy, finding community, and creating family. Coming out about your relationship style is a very serious decision, one that requires careful consideration. Finding others like you can help bring you support, friendship, resources, and understanding. Creating a chosen family of other nonmonogamous people builds a network of like-minded folks around you. Note that this chapter deals with the adults in your life. For information on raising children and coming out to them, see Chapter 17, Raising Children.

Benefits of Coming Out about Nonmonogamy

There are many reasons to come out about your open relationship. Probably one of the most obvious is that you can be open about all aspects of your life; you don't have to hide your lifestyle, lie about certain activities, withhold information, or sneak around. Coming out prevents misunderstandings and speculation; for example, if someone who doesn't know about your relationship style runs into you with a partner other than the one they know, they are likely to assume you're cheating, since cheating is much more prevalent and acknowledged than consensual nonmonogamy. This is a misinterpretation many nonmonogamous people despise, because their relationships are consensual. Coming out fits with a personal philosophy of openness: if you value honesty in relationships, you want that honesty to extend beyond romantic/love relationships. Sharing the whole picture with loved ones can feel like a weight lifted off your shoulders, but more important, it can deepen your intimacy with them.

Although most of their friends knew, married couple Josh and Andi decided to come out to their family as both bisexual and polyamorous after a few years of being polyamorous. "We felt that...the double life we were living with our family, the things that we had to keep from [them], didn't really jibe with our honesty and openness. And we weren't ashamed of what we were doing," Josh says. Andi says, "We stuck together when we decided to tell them because we thought that this was something we would continue for the rest of our lives... We didn't see it [as] a phase. We felt this is who we are. We identified so deeply with it."

Some respondents mentioned having to tell loved ones that additional partners were "friends," which wasn't the whole truth, and, in some cases, did not convey their importance in their lives. When you come out, people can know who your partners are and what they mean to you. Dillon came out to his family as both polyamorous and bisexual at Thanksgiving. He wanted to bring two of his partners home with him and didn't want to have to introduce one as just a friend. "As it turned out, my family was very supportive, and I think I was the person most nervous that Thanksgiving. It worked out beautifully because I was able to honor both of my lovers and honor my family too—they got to meet both of these amazing people in my life, and got to meet 'all of me' as well."

Coming out can also be an opportunity to educate those around you. Many people believe, erroneously, that they don't know anyone in a nonmonogamous relationship, and they make assumptions about people who are. Giving them the opportunity to get to know someone in an alternative relationship goes a long way toward understanding and acceptance. Lee says, "I don't wear a neon sign about it, but I don't take any measures to disguise anything, either. If I hear someone bashing nonmonogamy, [it] compels me to stand up as an example of responsible nonmonogamy that has lasted longer than the average mono/hetero pairing."

Risks of Coming Out

For some people, there are just as many reasons *not* to come out about their open relationship as there are for disclosing it. One of the most frequently cited—and a significant one—is that with children there is the potential for a custody dispute. When it comes to custody, in most parts of the country judges have considerable leeway in deciding who is a fit parent and who is not. Unfortunately, it is far more common for people in open relationships to lose custody of their children than for their nonmonogamy not to be an issue. Two of my interviewees lost custody of their children because they are polyamorous.

Others decided to be selective in coming out because of potential custody issues. Ginger has a 10-year-old daughter from a previous marriage who lives with her ex-husband, and a 3-year-old daughter with her current husband. She and her husband have not come out to the older child (whose custody they share), but the younger child, who lives with them, has known all along. One concern is that the 3-year-old might out them to the 10-year-old, who might tell her father, and he could challenge the current custody arrangement.

Daria, who's in a triad with a man and a woman, did not have a positive experience coming out to her mother: "My mom basically shut down for about three months. She couldn't handle anything more than [her] job and feeding herself... She gave me her perspective, and [told me] why I was a horrible person, why she did not agree with my choices... In an email, she wrote that she does not want any children we might have to be raised in this environment, and she would do her best to get custody of them." Because Daria plans to have children, she is very worried about her mother's threat to assume custody.

Another frequently cited reason for not coming out is the risk of losing one's job. Several people I interviewed or their partners work for government agencies or have high-profile jobs, and they fear negative repercussions. People who work with children believe their relationships will be misunderstood, seen as deviant and harmful to kids. One triad was concerned that a member might lose his security clearance if it was discovered he had a wife and a co-husband. Dani works as a minister in a Methodist Church: "I am not out at this church. It's a very conservative congregation. If I were at a different congregation, a little less conservative, and if they hadn't just run off their previous music director because he was gay, maybe I would be out. I hate not being out, but it's also self-preservation."

Whatever poly style you adopt, all nonmonogamous relationships are alternative relationships. They contradict most people's expectations, and many people are against any relationship other than monogamy for supposedly moral or religious reasons, or due to just plain ignorance and bigotry. Some people choose not to come out because of the stigma of nonmonogamous relationships and the fear of criticism or rejection from friends, family, and co-workers.

The hardest thing is living in a culture that doesn't sanction such relationships. That is, if one shares one's lifestyle with someone else, one may be labeled a "sex freak" or worse. —Dahlia

For some folks, where they live dictates how out they are to others. It's especially difficult for those who live in conservative communities. Ilana and Luke, who live in the Deep South, are out to almost no one about being polyamorous. Luke says:

> There are times when we would like to act according to our beliefs, but because of the prevailing belief system, we must be very circumspect in how we behave in public. This is sometimes difficult for us and causes feelings of disgust, resentment, and displeasure with society, especially here in the Bible Belt of the Deep South. People meddle, pry, condemn, evangelize, gossip.

They have consciously chosen not to date anyone in or near their hometown for fear of the gossip it could generate or potential problems if a partner (or ex) decided to out them. In addition, when partners from out of town come to visit, they must be very careful not to be affectionate in public:

> We've had a number of negative experiences of people who see things, make projections, say things to our friends, out us to our minister, so that's probably the most difficult part… But the second part is finding like-minded people, just to get along with, discuss issues and feelings with… We hardly have any friends here we can talk to about the issues involved with having multiple partners.

Deciding What's Right for You

There can be significant consequences in your life if you reveal you are not monogamous. You can be discriminated against at work or school, or when you seek housing or a job. Remember that there is no protection under the law for someone living in a committed triad, or for a polyamorous mother with four partners. Your open relationship can be used against you during a divorce, custody dispute, or other legal proceeding. You may be ostracized by your neighbors, social or political groups, your place of worship, and, perhaps most devastatingly, friends and family. As you weigh your options, consider these questions:

- How much does your open relationship affect your daily life?
- How might the people you love react to the announcement that you are nonmonogamous?
- How important is it that the following people know you are non-monogamous: family members, friends, co-workers, neighbors?
- How would you feel if you were rejected by family members, friends, co-workers, and neighbors?
- What kind of job do you have? Would being out put your job in jeopardy?
- Do you have children? Are there potential custody issues?
- What is the general social, political, and religious climate where you live?
- Do you have access to a local group of swingers, polyamorous people, or other folks in open relationships?
- Do you have a support system in case your coming out goes badly?

Your Coming Out

Once you have considered the potential consequences and risks, you still have plenty to think about if you decide to come out, including whom to come out to, how to come out, how to address people's concerns, and what to do if it doesn't go well.

Whom Should You Tell?

You don't have to come out to everyone in your life. In fact, being selective is often a necessary part of the process. You must carefully consider whom you're going to tell: immediate or extended family members, children, ex-partners or ex-spouses, friends, acquaintances, neighbors, employers, co-workers, employees, landlords, your lawyer, your doctors—think about all the people you have contact with who observe you in your relationship or with whom your relationship naturally comes up in conversation.

Make a preliminary list and sort everyone on it into categories. First up: who needs to know? This might be your children's teachers and school administrators so that co-parents have permission to pick them up from school; or your lawyer, who is drafting your wills. Next, whom do you want to tell? Think about friends, family, and co-workers. Finally, whom do you *not* want to tell? Perhaps you're happy to keep it from the town gossip, some neighbors, or even the house sitter. It's really up to you whom you decide to share this part of your life with.

How to Come Out and What to Expect

> *Our coming-out process has been very deliberate. We have tried to present our 'trilationship' [a triad of three men] in a time and space that allows people to ask questions, express concerns, and be heard. It has proven to be time-consuming.* —Turner

Turner's point is well taken: be prepared to dedicate a lot of time and energy to the people you come out to. Consider how you'd like to come out to a particular person. Depending on the relationship, a face-to-face sit-down may be the most appropriate. You want to approach the person with love, respect, and honesty; if you go into the talk feeling defensive or quick to respond to criticism, it will likely become confrontational. Be calm, speak your mind, then listen.

Many people choose to write a letter and follow it up in person. If you have a lot to say and aren't sure you will remember it all, writing a letter can help you say everything you intend to say, be as detailed as you like, and get all your points across. A letter allows the recipient to react in whatever way they want, take the time to digest the information, and come to terms with it before any discussion.

Whatever format you choose for making this announcement, keep in mind why you're coming out to this particular person. You might say, "I respect you and value your presence in my life. Our relationship is important enough to me that I want to be honest and share this significant part of my life with you. I am the same person you have known all along. This relationship choice may not be your cup of tea, but it works for me, and I'm happy. I hope you will respect my choice to live this way."

As part of your coming out, you must be clear about who else knows and whether discretion may be called for. If the person you come out to has questions, take the time to answer them as thoroughly as you can. Offer him a list of books, articles, or websites so he can better understand your open relationship. (See the Resource Guide for some suggestions.) Emphasize that you are available to help her process the information in whatever way she needs.

Positive coming-out experiences can be supportive, validating, and truly inspirational to people. When it goes well, there is cause for thanks and celebration. But you should be prepared for the possibility that coming out will be a negative experience. Several people discussed coming out to parents who are liberal, only to find that there was a double standard at work. For example, Meredith enjoys having political and intellectual conversations with her parents, and when she brought up the idea of plural marriage, her mother said, "As long as they're consenting adults, that's fine." But when she told them she was actually living in a triad, her parents changed their tune:

> [My mother] and my father didn't react very well. They told me, "The relationship is going to fall apart. You're doing a disservice to both young men. You're hurting them no matter what they say. The way you show you're committed is to be monogamous. You're hurting us, you're hurting them, you're gonna hurt yourself. The situation is gonna blow up."

Whom Are You Out To?

Here's a look at the people interviewees have come out to about their relationship style:

69% All friends

22% Selected friends

2% A few friends only

40% All family

27% Selected family

27% All co-workers

19% Selected co-workers

21% All friends, all family, and all co-workers

This kind of reaction, from parents who may be fine with open relationships in theory—for other people—but not for their children, is common. Remember that parents have certain expectations, wishes, and fantasies about who their children will grow up to be, and when you revise—or in their eyes, shatter—their expectations, it can be very difficult for even the most accepting parents. Aiden, who lives in a triad with two women in Phoenix, says, "[My parents] kind of accept this is who I am now. They raised me to be very accepting of other people and open-minded, so I have occasionally joked to my mom, when she's in a joking mood, 'You made me the way I am'... You know how people's parents are okay when someone else's kid is gay, but they get upset when it's their kid? That's how my parents were about the poly thing." If your parents are truly open-minded and committed to your happiness, they will likely come around with time and patience.

Coming out can be met with a barrage of harsh words, judgment, and criticism. Some people don't understand what open relationships are, and they may revert to common myths and misconceptions, like, "So you're a swinger? Is it like a big orgy at your house all the time?" You can respond to comments such as these with openness and clarification. Other people won't accept a relationship style that challenges their own or what they believe to be an acceptable model; their arguments against you may invoke religious or moral beliefs. If anyone judges you in this way, it's important to emphasize the consent and ethical nature of your relationship; stress that your chosen structure may not work for that person, but it works for you and your partners.

Other critics may lash out at you because of their own ambivalence or dissatisfaction with monogamy; they unconsciously envy what you're doing and wish they could do it too, but instead of saying so, they criticize you. It is nearly impossible to argue with people who are not in touch with their unacknowledged fears, desires, and motives. You may simply have to accept the unfavorable opinion that certain people express about your choice.

With some family members, no matter what you do, your coming out may not go as you'd like it to. Andi was a virgin when she married her husband, and she later came out as bisexual and polyamorous: "My siblings were all pretty cool with it, like, 'It's not really for me, but if you're happy…' My parents were very hurt by it. Like crying, depressed… [They are] Catholic, religious… I think they really worried about us and probably feared for our relationship. I think that they were disappointed in a way, and hurt."

Lena, 54, a legal secretary who lives in the Washington, DC, area, grew up in East Tennessee, where she was raised as a Southern Baptist. When she discovered polyamory and her bisexuality, she was thrilled to have found a new way of life that really worked for her. She was so happy about it she wanted to share it with her sister:

[My sister had] gone back to the Baptist Church and got heavily involved in religion in a way that was much more Holy Roller than it ever was when we were growing up. So I came out to her, and her response was "[My husband] and I are devastated by this. We think this is totally wrong. You shouldn't be doing this. I'm not going to tell you that you can't, but we can't talk to you about it. We don't want to hear about it, we don't want to know."... That was very hurtful, very hard, because she's my only sister. I'm still in touch with my family and we still get together at holidays, but I feel that I have to leave this huge part of my life behind when I visit them. I can't be me.

Although her mother was accepting, Lena learned a difficult lesson from her experience with her sister. She decided not to tell other family members whom she believed were less open and more bigoted than her sister.

Addressing People's Concerns

Be prepared for questions, concerns, and criticism from the people you come out to. It's a good idea to arm yourself with responses before the discussion takes place. Remember, no matter how outlandish or offensive their reaction, stay calm, don't become defensive, and offer a well-reasoned response. Below are some potential concerns and suggested responses. (You may want to review Chapter 2, Myths about Open Relationships, as well.)

Being nonmonogamous is not what God intended.
A poly Methodist minister had this to say: "I believe God created me who I am, with the needs that I have. And when I don't act out all of who I am, then I'm not only dishonoring myself, I'm dishonoring God. So for me, to be in a poly relationship that actually builds my faith and helps me be a better faith person and be a better minister is really answering who God is asking me to be."

I worry you're putting yourself in danger of STDs since you have so many sex partners.
My partners and I have been tested for everything, and we get tested regularly. In addition, I am very careful and always practice safer sex with partners I am not fluid-bonded with.

People who can't be monogamous have issues: you need therapy.
Everyone has issues concerning relationships; this is not about me not settling down with one person. Simply because I have made a different choice from yours doesn't mean I am screwed up.

You just haven't found the right person. When you do, you'll be monogamous.
I have found the right person! In fact, I've found three! Together they bring so much joy to my life.

Is this because your last marriage/relationship failed?
My last relationship taught me a lot about what I want and what makes me truly happy. I realized that I cannot expect one person to fulfill all my needs. I prefer to have multiple partners, since each relationship is unique and enriches the others.

This is going to destroy your relationship with your spouse/primary partner.
We communicate openly and honestly about our nonmonogamy. My other relationships enhance my primary relationship and take the pressure off it to be everything to me.

Some people object to your relationship style not for any specific reason but simply because, for them, it's wrong. Remember that people often criticize you when a decision you make doesn't reflect their values, or when it calls into question how they live their lives. Some people disapprove, some may feel threatened, and others might be envious (and unaware of it). Do not let anyone make you feel guilty. Remind them that these are *your* choices.

When Someone Outs You

When someone else outs you, you lose control of a significant step in your coming-out process—deciding whether and when to tell someone. But you can take charge of the situation. If someone outs you to a friend, family member, or co-worker, take the reins and address it immediately, even though the moment may not be ideal. Rather than focus on why you haven't come out already, direct your attention to giving the person clear information. Perhaps he has heard gossip or innuendo; set the record straight with as much detail as you feel comfortable sharing. If you discover you've been outed, seek support from friends, family, or a therapist who already knows about your relationship style. You may feel hurt, betrayed, or angry, but don't bring those emotions into your coming-out discussion. Remember, you have no reason to feel shame or guilt about your choices. Being pushed out is not fun, but once you're out, take a deep breath, hold your head high, and be ready to process the news with your loved ones.

Finding Community

During the coming-out process, obtaining support from people like yourself can be invaluable. They can answer questions, give you advice, and share their own experiences. Connecting with other people in open relationships is important not only when you're thinking about coming out. Finding like-minded people can help you feel less alienated and isolated, period. You can share your hopes and frustrations, and give and receive support, understanding, and validation. You can get help in figuring out what you want, negotiating agreements, and resolving relationship conflicts. When you find community, you also find friends and potential partners.

I was amazed to read how Joan and Larry Constantine found people to interview for their book *Group Marriage* in the early 70s. They began with members of an ad hoc, unnamed organization that hosted meetings in New England and published a newsletter titled *The Harrad Letter*. From there they followed vague leads and rumors as well as letters they received; they literally drove all over the country to find people living in multilateral marriages—many of whom were not open about their lifestyle and naturally suspicious of people who wanted to meet them.

Today, it's a lot easier to find people who are in nonmonogamous, swinger, polyamorous, polyfidelitous, mixed orientation, BDSM, and open relationships. The Internet has changed the way people locate information and each other, and there are plenty of websites, blogs, online forums and communities, and email Listservs that provide resources and support. While online support can be useful, it's also important to meet real people who are practicing nonmonogamy. I encourage you to do some research into local support groups, workshops, events, and conferences in your area. (Refer to the Resource Guide at the end of the book to get started.)

Families, Tribes, and Networks

During the past century, the dominant family structure has shifted from large, extended families with multiple generations living together to the smaller nuclear family; this shift has been well documented, along with its downside, including increased isolation and dependence on a smaller number of people. Some people who identify as polyamorous have reenvisioned the family as a chosen group of like-minded members rather than as a group that belongs together because of blood relation or marriage. These larger groups—consisting of four to 50 members—are called families, tribes, or networks. Although the use of the term *family* here overlaps with its meaning as used by some polyfidelitous groups, family in this sense is equivalent to extended family.

Relationships within a family can vary greatly and may include one's lovers, ex-lovers, partners, partners' partners, friends, biological family, children, and so on. What they have in common is that all members consider themselves bound to one another as part of a family. This larger network may have a name, be centered on a patriarch or matriarch, may encompass people from a specific geographic region, or be organized around a shared interest like BDSM. The level of regular contact between members within the network varies widely, but this is a chosen family whose members rely on one another for unconditional love, acceptance, help, friendship, and caretaking. They often come together for holidays, and support each other with childcare, a place to stay, or financial help. They join forces during major life changes such as the birth of a child, a major illness, or death.

Dillon, a bisexual man from New York, says, "While I have no problem with one-time-only sex, I prefer creating and sustaining relationships that include sex as a means of showing affection. I prefer being sexually affectionate and sensual in my friendships, and I have cultivated a large community of like-minded, similarly expressive people. We occasionally have group get-togethers that include sex, and we play with whom we please, with fervor and glee, according to where people are at in the moment. To some this might seem like 'casual sex,' but I take my friendships and sexual expression seriously. Both are very important to me and feed and nurture me greatly." It is important to Dillon that all his partners know each other and that they become friends; as a result, he has created an extended network of over 40 people, made up of friends, lovers, partners, partners of partners, and others with whom he has a relationship of some kind. "That is how I live my life these days… Everybody knowing each other and meeting each other's partners is how, for me, I think it all works… We have this network that is actually healthy and kind of like a family because we don't hide it."

Jimmy is part of a queer leather family in Pittsburgh, most of whose 12 members are polyamorous. It originated in the mid-nineties, growing out of a local S/M organization: "Some of our members don't live in Pittsburgh. Some lived here and moved. Some never lived here. Some don't play any longer, but everybody is on board, accepting each other's perversions and tastes and needs and quirks." Jimmy explains how he sees them as a family rather than a group of friends:

> In a group of friends, everyone really likes each other and they have things in common. When there's a fight or someone takes on something that others don't agree with, you get dropped from the circle. You get married, you leave the circle, and that's often the way your friends work. In our group…there's always someone in the family that you don't like so much, but you have some kind of bond with them. You still consider them yours, even if you don't like them. I'm not saying I don't like them… I'm saying…you celebrate all the birthdays, all the holidays. When someone's in the hospital, you arrange to take out the dog and things like that. We do the things that families do… We've had people go through issues and into therapy, we've had people divorce, we've had people partner with nonleather folk, and we've worked out how those people can stay within the family.

In his interview, Jimmy stressed that his leather family was a big part of his polyamorous identity: "Our commitment as a family is as strong, important, and valuable as the individual relationships I have."

Some groups are more loosely organized, like Brett's: "Our tribe, based in Seattle, includes two of my wife's lovers, two of my co-husband's lovers, and a large number of people we consider family. We have been attached to them for over 10 years. I consider them tertiary partners, but we do make time in our lives to spend with them."

The notion of chosen family came up a lot in my interviews, even among folks who are not part of larger networks, like Brett, Jimmy, and

Dillon. There was plenty of talk among polyamorous people about how they considered their partners—however many there were—to be like a family. Aiden sees his triad as a family and relates his desire to live with more than one person to his upbringing:

> My family was a big extended family. My aunts and uncles and cousins were always around. It was a very warm feeling, very "We got your back." I like that, and I think that leans toward why I draw multiple people around me now.

While he appreciates his family of origin, Aiden makes it clear that his new, chosen family will make medical decisions for him. This is significant, because he has multiple disabilities and is currently in a wheelchair:

> If anything happens to me, my bois get to make the decisions, not my biological family. My birth family knows this, and though they were a bit hurt at first, they have come to realize that the bois are my family just as much as my parents and sister. [They] are relieved I have such a tight-knit, loving family to live happily with, care for, and be cared for by.

In their 1973 book *Group Marriage*, Larry and Joan Constantine noted some of the benefits of multiperson marriages they discovered in their research:

> In other ways, voluntary intimate networks can fulfill many of the functions of extended families and close communities providing, for example, alternate resources for temporary needs. Based on choice and involving families in similar stages of the family life cycle, intimate networks can avoid some of the tensions and resented obligations of the extended families based on blood ties.[1]

For people in alternative relationships, *family* is a significant word that conjures up two groups of people: the families we come from and the families we create for ourselves. The concept of a chosen family has been researched and described by social scientists. As nonmonogamous and polyamorous people redefine what it means to be spouses, partners, and lovers, they are also redefining family. In the next chapter we will turn our attention to another aspect of family: raising children.

PROFILE: JUDY AND TRAVIS

"It's been a new beginning for both of us in many ways."

JUDY AND TRAVIS, both in their late 50s, have been married for 35 years. They are teachers and live together in New York. Six years ago, Judy discovered an interest in BDSM, and she shared her desire with Travis: "I'd kept quiet about it for so long. I wanted to build in success and have him respond well and not argue, so it was a long conversation. I showed him things I'd been reading about safety, etc. I tried to enlist him with some light play, and he did try, but it didn't work at all. Realizing that he couldn't provide me with this, I told him that I had to explore this, I was going to find someone, and I refused to sneak around. He was okay—not jumping up and down for joy or anything—but okay. He said, 'Just don't do anything stupid.'"

When she made her disclosure to him, Travis had already discovered he was gay, but he was in the closet: "Here I am, a closeted gay man, and Judy's finding this outlet… It would be in my best interest to just simply listen, not fly off the handle. In some ways, I was relieved that she had found something that was the path that she needed to take."

At that point in their relationship, their sex life "was nonexistent for the most part," but Judy believed she could explore BDSM without sex. "He even asked me if it would involve sex, and I said maybe… I didn't really think it would, though, but once I had an experience, I realized that I couldn't do it without sex. I didn't tell him when I actually started having sex with a partner. I didn't go into details. He doesn't want to hear the details, even now."

Judy had begun to suspect that Travis was gay. She asked him, but he denied it. "He really couldn't come out. I kept opening doors for him, holding them open…but he couldn't walk through. I think that since so many wives respond so negatively and he'd heard such horror stories, he was still afraid to let me know. I now know he was doing things behind my back—and here I was open about my life."

Travis finally came out to her about a year after she began seeing other people. He admits that before his coming out, he did "the usual sneaking around and stuff which I'm not particularly proud of." They agreed that splitting up was unnecessary. "One, we love each other," Judy says. "We are very much in tune, artistically, and are really best friends. We have a beautiful daughter whom we both adore, and while we didn't mention it, splitting up after being married so long would be a *huge* hassle and financially very uncomfortable."

Judy admits that the timing was also important: "I also had a regular partner I was seeing, having more sex and play than I ever thought possible…so it was a good time to tell me. If he'd told me when I wasn't getting any and not in a happy place, I can't honestly say how I would have reacted." Travis says, "Once I was out, once we were out to each other, then it became this interesting situation…it was kind of non-threatening… The uniqueness about it is that she has chosen her path in what is essentially an alternative lifestyle and mine is alternative as well. But then, they don't necessarily conflict with one another because I'm not seeking, let's say, another woman or a relationship that's heterosexual."

When they came out to their daughter, they came out together— Judy's interest in BDSM, Travis's sexual orientation, and their open relationship. "She is incredibly proud to have us as parents; apparently our 'cool factor' went up. Many of her friends come from homes where parents are divorced and angry. As she says, we put the fun back in dysfunctional."

After coming out, Travis explored his sexuality and had some casual partners before meeting his current boyfriend. Surprisingly, he did not have a tough time explaining that he was married: "My boyfriend, he's seen it all, essentially, every possible combination of open relationships... My situation is not necessarily a problem for him because he understands and he's got this openness about him anyway. He likes the idea that he and I have been able to carve out this kind of relationship that's healthy and stable and sexually active and honest and Judy is kind of a part of it." Travis and his boyfriend have been together for a year and a half, and they are monogamous.

Judy has casual play partners, but no one steady or serious. Travis says, "I communicate often and regularly with my wife. It is the only way to survive any relationship. I have unfortunately learned that rather late in life but I'm working on it... Because the relationship with my wife is rather unusual and untraditional, we find that we are constantly making rules and redefining them, as we need to. With my gay partner, it is pretty much ditto—we make the rules and live by them until we feel the need to reevaluate, and then sit down and revamp them as needed."

"Last Christmas, I invited my husband's beau to visit," Judy says. "I had met him twice before, but he'd never stayed very long. I wanted him to know that he was welcome in our family. He is an absolutely lovely man, fits in very well—he and I even trade emails regularly. He loves to help out in the kitchen, and I welcome him, even though he's terrible at washing dishes. Christmas night, my husband leaned in to give me a kiss and whispered, 'Thanks for being so wonderful.' That was a great gift." Travis says, "Think about it—your wife, your daughter, and your gay boyfriend all laughing and opening up presents on Christmas morning. Fabulous! Talk about accepting and sharing."

"For me, our coming out...didn't open up my sex life, it gave me one," Judy says. "Arguing about not having sex is a terrible way to live. It opened my life, and I really think Travis saw—and was moved to open his. It has opened up our lives, created more communication, and an even deeper relationship. It erased the fear. It has seemed to have an effect on our entire life." Travis agrees that it has strengthened their existing connection: "We have this strong, loving relationship of thirty-some-odd years of being together. We know how each other thinks, how each other acts and reacts in certain ways; we're comfortable with each other. [Our coming out] has taken us apart in some ways, but it's also brought us back together. Our discussions have never been more honest, funnier, more enjoyable. We can speak absolutely openly to each other... We all need somebody in our life we can say anything to and not be judged."

Chapter 17

Raising Children

IN AN ARTICLE on being a polyamorous parent, Valerie White writes: "Human babies are wired for clans, not 'nuclear families' where mom is home alone with the kids. Therefore, I believe that raising children in ways that are healthy and natural for them is one thing polyamory can be good at."[1] Valerie is a 62-year-old attorney from Massachusetts. She lives with her primary partner and husband, Ken, and his partner, Judy. Valerie and Ken have several children and Ken and Judy have two. "Ken and I were present during Judy's labor and delivery of the twins. I helped to nurse them. We are three equal co-parents. Judy would probably not have decided to have children if there hadn't been three of us—and me an experienced parent."

In a reader survey conducted by *Loving More* magazine in 2002, 26 percent of 1,000 respondents had children under 18 living with them. Among my interviewees, 50 have children (not necessarily under 18 or living with them). One of the benefits of raising children in a polyamorous household is that everyone has more help: there are more adults to meet the needs of each child. Lee, who raises a toddler with his primary partner in San Francisco, concurs:

When there were three of us involved, sharing each other and the burdens of parenting, I felt that the benefits of nonmonogamy were really coming through for me. If two of us needed a date, one of us could be the one to stay at home with the child. We had a few instances where we all wanted date time, so we each took two hours of "rearing time" to allow the other two "pairing time."

With more pairs of hands changing diapers, helping with homework, and driving to soccer practice, multipartner households, like extended families, alleviate some of the burdens on the traditional nuclear family. But polyamorous people who parent do more than raise their children: they help redefine what constitutes a family.

Benefits and Risks of Coming Out to Children

Coming out about your relationship style to your children is a complex but important decision. Among my interviewees with children, 52 percent have come out to them and 11 percent have come out to their older children—a much higher rate than found in other research.

A 1982 study by Watson and Watson found that while 75 percent of polyamorous survey respondents wanted their children to know of their lifestyle, only 21 percent had actually informed their children of the full extent of their involvements with other partners. "Some include their children in the company of their secondary partners, and indicate that they enjoy the process of modeling an alternative for their children. Other parents feel that sharing the news of their lifestyle would be too upsetting for their children, or would not be understood, or would be shared haphazardly with neighbors and school friends."[2]

Just as there are pros and cons to coming out to adults, there are benefits and risks of coming out to children. Whether your children live with you part-time or full-time, whether you see them frequently or infrequently, they are a big part of parents' lives. Children are often more observant, intuitive, and knowledgeable about the world around them than we give them credit for. At some point, children are apt to figure out that a parent has a nontraditional relationship; coming out to them puts it right out on the table and creates a forum for them to ask questions and get answers.

Being honest about your relationship(s) can foster a sense of openness and candor in your relationship with your kids. You don't have to offer false explanations about the identity of someone in your life, withhold affection for someone in their presence, or otherwise cover up your relationships. Being up front also sends a clear message: your relationship choices are valid and acceptable rather than shameful or something to hide. In an essay on poly parents, John Ullman extends this to sex as well: "Attempting to cover up our polyamory would only send a message that sex was surrounded by anxiety and hypocrisy, and perhaps we did things we were ashamed of."[3]

Alongside the benefits of honesty and sharing are some significant concerns. Some people wonder if their nontraditional relationship will confuse or psychologically damage their kids. There is limited research on children raised by polyamorous parents. As part of their 1973 study of multilateral marriage, Joan and Larry Constantine collaborated with Angela Hunt, a professor and child psychology specialist from Iowa State University, to conduct a substudy of the children of such marriages. They concluded:

> On most issues, the structure of the family has little bearing on the children's development. What does affect them is the nature and the quality of their parents' interactions with them and with each other. As in nuclear families, good marriages are good for children, bad marriages are not.[4]

More recently, in the magazine *Proud Parenting*, licensed clinical social worker Arlene Istar Lev declared: "I want to be blatantly clear, at the risk of upsetting my more conservative readers, that a polyamorous

According to the *Loving More* Polyamory Survey (2002)

- 26 percent of respondents had children under 18 living with them
- 13.3 percent had experienced discrimination by Child Protective Services because of a poly relationship
- 61 percent had adopted or would be open to adopting children within a poly relationship[5]

lifestyle can be a healthy, loving, nurturing environment in which to raise children, regardless of one's sexual orientation, marital status, or methods of conception."[6]

Just as with coming out to adults, it is a valid concern that children may not be accepted or may be ostracized by their peers and others in your community. If your custody of the children could be challenged by a disapproving social worker, co-parent, ex-spouse, or grandparent, your open relationship could be used against you.

What to Consider Before You Tell Them

There are several issues to consider before your tell your kids about your open relationship. First, how much does your relationship style affect their daily lives? This will determine how much they need to know. For example, if you are a solo polyamorist, you can simply say that you date multiple people who know about each other. If you practice partnered nonmonogamy, additional partners could be introduced as friends, which would be honest and appropriate. However, if you're part of a triad, have several long-term poly partners, or live with (or plan to live with) multiple partners, your children will have more contact with partners and more chances to see you interact. Explaining the nature of your relationships can be much more important in these cases.

Another issue to consider is how mature your children are. The nature of the information you give them should be age-appropriate and suitable to their level of maturity. You should also assess the community in which you live. If the social climate is not supportive, there will be a bigger burden on your children to field questions and criticism. George and his two triad partners are raising two daughters. He noticed that there was more speculation and questioning when they lived in a conservative suburb than when they moved to the city:

> *Before we moved back down to the city, when we were living in the suburbs, Suzanne, our older daughter, certainly did have more [of] her peers [ask] "What's up with your family?" Our kids don't wonder why their family is different, but other kids do. Suzanne says, "This is what it is, this is who my family is." The kids are a little more disposed to say "okay" but then they'll go and talk to their parents. If anyone has an issue, it's the other children's parents... If our kids have had any kind of extracurricular friendships with other kids, either their parents are open-minded enough just to not let it faze them or they're closed-minded in the passive-aggressive Minnesota way—they just kind of recede into the background.*

How to Tell Them

If you decide to tell your children, set aside some dedicated time to talk to them about it; be prepared to spend as much or as little time as they want. Be proactive and confident when you approach the subject; if you're anxious about the conversation, your kids will sense it and it might make them uneasy. Do not make assumptions about what they know or don't know; tell them everything you intend to tell them, and if they already know some of it, let them reveal that. Explain the details in age-appropriate language; a 16-year-old can understand the term *polyamory*, but it won't mean anything to a 4-year-old. Depending on your level of openness with them, leave sex out of the discussion, or minimize it. Put your relationship in context for them; if they know other kids who have gay and lesbian parents, single parents, or step-parents, offer them as examples of families like yours. Aaron, a computer engineer from Minneapolis, has two daughters and lives in a triad:

> *We live in a fairly progressive community: [our children] know gay people, a lesbian couple who have kids, people who have divorced and remarried… So there are all varieties of mixed families around us. When we got together, we sat down with Gwen, our older daughter, and said, Hey, this is what's going on. Then, when [our partner] Penny not just moved in but we all got married, we said, This is what's going on, this is a part of our family. [Our younger daughter] Bonnie was actually born after we were in a relationship with Penny. She gets that we have a different family, home life, and relationship than most other kids do. But I don't know if she's tried to figure it out; it's more like, That's what you have, this is what I have.*

When kids hear something about their parents, they want to know how it will affect *them* and *their lives*. Reassure them that you love them, your partners love them, and no one is breaking up or having secret affairs. If you are no longer involved with one of your children's parents, assure your child that your other partners do not intend to replace their mom or dad. Emphasize that each adult cares deeply about them and is there for them. Explain that while your family may not look like other people's families, that's what it is: a family.

Sandra is part of a five-person circle, four of whom live together and are raising four children together: "We explained it to them according to their understanding, in whatever age-appropriate terms we could figure out. It was never a 'secret' from them, and we let them know we loved each other very much and wanted to expand our family."

Diane and Mike live with their triad partner, Derek, who is divorced. Among them they have 10 kids, seven who live with them. Diane says:

> *The youngest don't know exactly what the relationship is but they always call Derek their second dad. The oldest know exactly what's going on. They don't care... Whenever one of the younger ones decides to ask me, I'm going to just tell her, it's like this: We have a very special relationship and it's not very often in life that you get to find somebody else to love this much. This is how we've been living and what's been going on this whole time. We don't love you any less and we don't love you any more. We just do the best we can with you. That's pretty much what we told the older kids.*

Once you tell your children, an important issue that you need to address with them is how and when to share this new information with others. This is one of the trickiest elements of coming out to kids. You want to make it clear that you are being open and honest, that your family is "just another kind of family," that you're telling them this because it is nothing to hide or keep secret. But in certain cases you have to tell them not to tell other people. While this sends a mixed message, it may be necessary if you live in an unsupportive community or if there could be career repercussions for one of your partners. You'll have to set ground rules about the people this information can be shared with, and you'll have to explain that there are people in the world who are ignorant and bigoted and don't understand other kinds of families. As part of this, ensure that your kids have someone to talk to about their feelings besides you; give them the option of seeing a therapist, and make sure to find one who has experience with people in alternative relationships.

For kids who were born into multipartner households, being part of a nontraditional family is all they know. It's not until they meet other kids that they realize their family is different. But this doesn't mean they won't have questions. Be prepared to sit down with them and have a conversation. Diane's older kids came to her first:

> Derek's kids [from his previous marriage] had told my older two kids. So they came to me, and I said, "Well, what do you know?" They explained to me what they knew. I told them they only had it half right because they thought that we were all just swingers. I said, "No. Do you notice how long Derek has lived with us?"... My oldest said, "Why is Derek still hanging around?" I told him the reason he's hanging around is because he loves you guys, as much as your dad or I do... That's why he makes you do your chores, watches you do your homework, goes to the zoo with us, you know, everything.

Cat is a 38-year-old massage therapist from central Oklahoma. She has two sons:

> Holt is 16 and Patrick is 8. Holt is quite aware, though I don't think he really knows or even cares which of my close friends are lovers and which are not. Patrick is somewhat aware but pays little or no attention. When they are here, they are among this big community of people of all ages and genders and lovestyles and nobody can really tell who's just being affectionate with a 'family' member and who's cuddling with a sweetheart. Their father and I divorced when Holt was 9 and Patrick was 18 months old. Holt had already been aware of our polyamory for several years, and his dad and new stepmom were together for some time before he and I split up. We were always very up front with Holt about our belief that people should be able to love as many people as they love... I answer Patrick's questions matter-of-factly. If he asks, "Why do you go on dates with girls and boys?" I say, "Because I love those people and I want to spend time with the people I love."

Ginger and her husband are polyamorous and have a daughter together who has grown up with their lifestyle: "She's grown up in a poly house, so she's knocked on the bedroom door and seen someone in bed with us on Saturday morning, but it's just like a kid who would climb into bed with their parents, which she's done her whole life." However, Ginger also has an older daughter who lives with her ex-husband, and that daughter doesn't know:

> I would be very comfortable talking about being poly with my [older] daughter. We have much better communication...than I had with my own mom. But I'm concerned about what her dad's reaction would be. I don't think it's okay to say, "I'm telling you this and you can't tell your father."... I want her to know she has a choice between monogamy and responsible nonmonogamy. But how can I do that without giving my ex a big gun to use against me if he wants to revisit custody at some point in the future? Waiting until a 10-year-old is 18 is surely not the answer. I don't want this to be a secret.

She is also concerned that at some point the younger daughter will out them to the older daughter inadvertently. It's a dilemma she continues to struggle with.

Practical Issues

Parents must interact with all sorts of institutions, organizations, and groups while raising children, including people involved with childcare programs, schools, sports teams, extracurricular activities, religious groups, and camps, not to mention teachers, health care providers, counselors, and others. It's important to establish who is an emergency contact and who has the right to pick up the child, make decisions, and sign forms.

When meeting with school officials and others, it's not always necessary to say "We are polyamorous," or "I have two husbands."

Instead, meet with them together and make the simple declaration, "We are Sunny's parents." In this age of queer parents, blended families, stepparents, and other alternative families, school administrators have grown familiar with the idea of children having more than two parents. George and his triad partners are out to many people, including those who interact with their children on a regular basis: "We've been pretty lucky with people not really blinking too much. I think it's because there's so much divorce and remarriage. The idea that there's a child who has two separate family units—a primary mother and father and another family unit [is not unheard of]. It just so happens we all live together and we're all still together. There are actually ways in which that ends up making it a little bit easier for us."

PROFILE: SANDRA, DOUG, RICK, GABRIELLE, AND JOAN

"We are a closed circle of five."

TWENTY-THREE YEARS AGO, Sandra met Rick, who was in an open relationship and was the first person to introduce her to the idea of nonmonogamy. He and Sandra dated for a while, Rick got married, and they continued to date. Then they lost touch for 12 years. When they found each other again, Sandra had met and married Doug, and Rick was married to Gabrielle. Sandra and Rick reconnected and realized they were still in love with each other. Sandra said, "I didn't want to mess up my marriage and I didn't want to mess up my relationship with [Rick] either. I said under no circumstances are we going to have an affair. But I don't know how to do this. We need to figure this out."

She had also been having some difficulties with her husband and they were in counseling, so she and Rick decided they'd just be friends. "It sounded almost impossible to do, because it was clear that we were more than friends and we really loved each other. We kept getting

closer and closer and then backing off." She decided to take a year off
from having any contact with Rick, work on her relationship with her
husband, then come back together and see what things looked like.
"During that year off, my husband and I worked on stuff and I explained
to him that I didn't think it was just about this other guy, I thought it
was about who I am as a person, my nature as a polyamorous person."
Her husband, Doug, gave her permission to see other people, and she
started dating; Doug began corresponding with Rick's wife, Gabrielle,
because she too was having issues with her spouse (Rick) being polyamorous. Doug and Gabrielle got to like each other and found they had
a lot in common. At one point, back in touch, Sandra asked Rick, "Are
our spouses falling in love with each other? How interesting is that!"

Four months into the year off, Doug and Gabrielle came to Sandra
and Rick and said, "Let's sit down and have a discussion about what this
is going to look like if we try this. If we're going to have a relationship
that would be polyamorous, what does everybody need?" The four of
them spent a weekend figuring out details such as physical and emotional safety, STDs, and veto power. "We hammered out all these things
without any guidelines at all, except somebody found a book called
Love without Limits," Sandra says. After the talk, they all decided to get
HIV tests. That night, Doug and Gabrielle had sex for the first time.

The couples, who lived four hours apart, began commuting to
spend time together. After a year, Sandra says, "Both the husbands
traveled quite a bit. Gabrielle was trying to raise her two kids and
homeschool them, and take care of her father with dementia. I was
trying to raise my two kids and go to school full-time. We just looked
at each other and went, 'This is stupid, why aren't we living together so
there are at least two parents home most of the time?'" So they bought
a house and all moved in together.

Shortly after they moved in, Rick announced that he wanted to
pursue a woman, Joan, from his past whom he had recently reconnected
with. The other three were wary but gave him permission; Rick and

Joan started dating. Sandra was having an especially hard time with it, so she flew to the East Coast to meet Joan, and, unexpectedly, an attraction between the two women developed. Joan divorced her estranged husband and became part of the group. Joan still lives on the East Coast and visits every two months. She has talked about eventually moving, but for now her career keeps her where she is. They all consider themselves a closed circle of five; however, Joan is closest to and has a sexual relationship with Sandra and Rick. Sandra says, "Joan has a hard time with being far away. She feels a little marginalized, but she realizes that it's her choice. I feel that I rearranged my entire life to make it possible to live with these people, and she's not willing to make that choice right now."

While the five are committed to one another, four of them are connected on a different level through daily living, a shared household, finances, and the children they co-parent, so there is definitely the sense of a quad within the five-person circle. The quad has a legal contract that delineates what percentage of the house each married couple owns and what share of household expenses they are responsible for. One of the stipulations of the contract is that it renews every seven years unless somebody objects.

Sandra has now been married to Doug for 23 years; the quad has been together for 12 years and the circle of five for a decade. Sandra and Doug have two daughters who are now 15 and 19. Rick and Gabrielle have two sons who are now 25 and 21. When the quad got together, the kids were 13, 10, 7, and 3. "They kind of just took it in stride," Sandra says:

> My youngest daughter [is] a very intuitive young person, very emotionally in tune with people. She kept saying to Rick, "Don't touch my mom." She knew something was up, something made her uncomfortable. The first time she burst into the bedroom first thing in the morning and she jumped on her dad and his other

partner, we weren't sure what was going to happen. She said,
"Oh, is that Gabrielle?" And he said, "Yeah." She said, "Okay."
We explained things as they could understand them.

When the oldest son was 16, Sandra says he called a meeting with
all five adults and said, "Look, I think what you're doing is wrong. It's
been really confusing for me, as I develop my sexuality. I need to get
out of this house, this situation, which means I'm moving out of town.
I want to let you know that's why I'm doing it. I need to get out on my
own and figure things out for myself." He had graduated from high
school early, so he moved out. Sandra says, "It was kind of hard for all
of us to hear that from him in the moment. Here he's making a judgment about us and our choice of lifestyle. Yet, at the same time, at the
end of that same conversation he said, 'But I want to let you know that
I love you all, and I just need to do this for myself.'

"It was painful for us at the moment that it took place, but in
hindsight we went, 'Hey, wait a minute, I could never have had that
conversation with my parents.' We did a good job. We were able to
give him the upbringing whereby he was able to have this really difficult conversation with five parents… After he had that little blowup,
he did go off on his own for about six months and then he came back,
and he continued to come back about twice a year and stay with us.
He finally moved out on his own, found his own place, and he still
loves us all and he still calls on us individually depending on what he
needs."

The other son is in college and still lives at home. "He's said to us
that the best thing he's gained from this is a couple of sisters he would-
n't have had, and he really liked having more siblings." Ultimately,
Sandra believes, growing up with polyamorous parents has helped
them mature and given them options for their future relationships:
"The youngest kids grew up with it and have been very comfortable
with it all along because it's been the norm for them. As they get into

their adult and sexuality years, they understand that some people love more than one person and sometimes that works out and sometimes it doesn't work out, it just depends on who the people involved are. I don't know if they're more emotionally mature, but [these kids] are as emotionally mature as any people their age, possibly more, because they've had different experiences."

Chapter 18

Safer Sex and Sexual Health

WHILE IT MAY NOT BE FUN, spontaneous, or sexy to some people, talking about your sexual history and health is crucial for everyone in relationships, and that's especially true for people who have multiple sexual partners. Defining your needs around sexual health and safety is a critical boundary that should be discussed, agreed to, and respected. It's important to arm yourself with as much information as you can about sexual health to make the most informed decisions. Remember: fucking without anxiety and doubt is sexy. In this chapter, I cover safer sex practices as well as the most common sexually transmitted infections in America, their symptoms, and their treatments.

While most people are probably familiar with the term *sexually transmitted disease*, or *STD*, in recent years medical professionals have adopted the term *sexually transmitted infection*, or *STI*, to better describe the realities of infection transmission. The difference is this: an STD is identified only when symptoms appear, but an STI is an infection before and after it causes symptoms. In other words, people can pass STIs to others even when they don't show any symptoms.

Safer Sex

Every sexual encounter we have with another person carries physical and emotional risks, responsibilities, and rewards. While you may not be able to anticipate or guard against feelings or psychological issues that arise from an erotic experience, you can do your best to protect your body from infection and disease. It's important to know what STIs are, how they are transmitted, and how to protect yourself from them. It's equally important for you and your partner(s) to get tested regularly for STIs.

Practicing safer sex can decrease the chances of STI transmission. Making informed decisions about safer sex with partners is a critical issue for people involved in nonmonogamous relationships of all kinds; safer sex was the one issue universally discussed in the interviews I conducted for this book. Even people who stated they had no rules when it came to their style of nonmonogamy talked about the importance of STI testing and safer sex. Most interviewees who have one or more long-term partners decided to become *fluid-bonded* with them. Being fluid-bonded mean you have unprotected sex with each other and regularly come into contact with each other's bodily fluids, including semen, vaginal secretions, and female ejaculate.

There are several different ways to set up safer sex:

- You practice safer sex with every partner.
- You are fluid-bonded with one partner and practice safer sex with all other partners.
- You are fluid-bonded with multiple partners in a group unit (like a triad or quad) and practice safer sex with all other partners.
- You are part of a fluid-bonded chain and practice safer sex with all partners outside the chain.

Several of the folks I interviewed are links in a fluid-bonded chain, the last option in the list above. It looks something like the diagram below. (Not an actual group; the names are fictitious.)

John + Jocelyn
    ||
    Bill + Barbara
        ||
Shelley + Sue

John is married to Jocelyn and is fluid-bonded with her. Jocelyn plays with a couple, Bill and Barbara, with whom she is also fluid-bonded. (Therefore, whether John plays with them or not, he is fluid-bonded with them as well.) Bill has sex with Shelley and Sue, another fluid-bonded couple. To create a safer sex chain, the six people sit down together, get tested, and when everyone tests negative for STIs, they agree that anyone can have unprotected sex with anyone else in the chain. They also agree that each person must practice safer sex with anyone outside the chain.

People set up a chain to become fluid-bonded with multiple others, but the more links are added to the chain, the more people you must trust with your sexual health. If one person slips up, everyone is affected. For example, if Sue has unprotected sex with someone whose STI status she doesn't know and then has sex with Shelley, giving her an infection, it can make its way back to John, even though Sue and John don't have sex. If you choose to become fluid-bonded with one or more partners, you should all abstain from unprotected sex for at least two weeks, get tested for all STIs, and continue to have only pro-tected sex—with all partners—while waiting for the results. Once you know you are negative for all STIs, you may begin having unprotected sex within the group while continuing to have safer sex with all other partners.

While every person I interviewed for this book mentioned fluid bonding, safer sex, or both, their definitions of "safer sex" varied greatly when I asked them to elaborate. It's important that you be rigorously specific when discussing these issues with your partner(s). You and your partner(s) can define safer sex in any way you like, but do not assume that when you say "I practice safer sex," or "I'd like us both to practice safer sex," the term has the same meaning for your partner that it does for you. Here are some examples of the safer sex guidelines given by interviewees:

- Condoms for vaginal and anal intercourse, no barriers for anything else
- Condoms for vaginal and anal intercourse, no barriers for oral sex, no ejaculation in fellatio
- Condoms for vaginal and anal intercourse, condoms for fellatio, dams for analingus, no barriers for cunnilingus
- Condoms for vaginal and anal intercourse, condoms for fellatio, dams for analingus, dams for cunnilingus only if the woman has her period
- Condoms for vaginal and anal intercourse, condoms for fellatio, dams for analingus and cunnilingus, gloves for manual penetration, condoms for sex toys

Guidelines for safer sex change as new research emerges about STI transmission, so negotiating safer sex should be an ongoing part of your discussion about nonmonogamy. Here are some of the tools you can use to protect yourself and your partners.

Gloves

Wearing a glove for external stimulation, penetration with fingers, and hand jobs protects both you and your partner, especially if you have any cuts, scratches, or even torn cuticles, which can provide direct access to your bloodstream for an STI. Gloves made of latex are the most popular and widely available, and latex is a good safer sex barrier. If, however, you are allergic or sensitive to latex, there are gloves made of other materials, including nitrile, vinyl, and neoprene. Powdered gloves are easier to get on and off, but the powder can irritate people's skin; if your skin feels itchy or turns red and you know you're not allergic to the glove material, find one that's not powdered.

Gloves come in several different sizes, from extra small to extra large, and it's important to find the right size for your hand. A glove that's too small will cut off your circulation and has a greater risk of tearing. One that is too big can feel uncomfortable to the receptive partner and gives the wearer less sensitivity. Besides being great for safer sex, gloves can make penetration smoother and more comfortable, especially if your nails are not perfectly trimmed and filed or if you have long nails.

Oral Sex Barriers

To protect yourself and your partner during cunnilingus and analingus, you can use one of several safer sex barriers. The most popular is a latex dental dam. Originally, safer sex practitioners coopted squares of latex designed for use by dentists (as the name indicates). Because they were not developed with sex in mind, dental dams are too small and too thick to make them ideal. Several companies—like Glyde, Slicks, Lixx, and Good Vibrations—have improved upon the dental dam, designing larger, thinner dams specifically for oral sex that do the job much better. Hot Dam makes polyurethane dams for those allergic to latex. Some dams come scented or flavored, and most are available at better sex toy stores.

To make your own dam out of a latex or nonlatex condom, you can cut an unlubricated condom up one side; these tend to be thinner, like Glydes, allowing both partners more feeling and greater sensitivity. You can also transform a latex glove into a dam: cut the wrist and the fingers off, leaving the thumb intact, then cut up the side where the pinkie was. Open it up, stick your tongue in the thumb slot, and voilà—it's like a condom for your tongue! This is my favorite kind of dam because it affords both giver and receiver the highest sensitivity.

For obvious reasons, it's best to use a glove that isn't powdered or to rinse the powder off before you put your mouth near it. Try putting a dab of lube on the inside and outside of the thumb for even more sensitivity.

Store-bought plastic wrap (brands like Saran Wrap) is not just for leftovers—it also makes a good barrier for cunnilingus and analingus. Plastic wrap is less expensive and easier to find than latex dams, which makes it more convenient. Another advantage: it can cover a lot more surface area and no one has to hold the dam in place. Try wrapping your sweetie's privates in plastic—think of it as a homemade thong for safe, hands-free licking. You can simply cut it off when you're all done.

For fellatio, you can use a flavored condom or an unlubricated condom. Condoms made for intercourse often come prelubed, and chances are you're not going to like the taste of the lube. Flavored condoms are made especially for oral sex, or you can use an unlubricated condom and add a dab of flavored lube or a lube you don't mind the taste of. To increase sensitivity, add a dab of lube to the inside of the condom before you put it on.

Condoms

Because of the concentration of STIs in semen (and precum) and the delicacy of the cervix and vaginal and rectal tissue, unprotected intercourse is among the riskiest of activities for the transmission of STIs. When used correctly and consistently, condoms are highly effective in preventing STI transmission; *correctly* is the key word here. There are more untrustworthy people than there are untrustworthy condoms. Three factors ensure a condom's effectiveness: proper fit, proper installation, and proper removal. Fit is incredibly important not only for the sensitivity of both partners, but also for safety. A condom that fits well is less likely to slip off or to break. Each brand of condom fits penises slightly differently. Brands like Exotica and LifeStyles make "snugger fit" styles, which are smaller than regular condoms. Popular larger size brands include Durex XXL, Kimono Maxx, LifeStyles XL, and Trojan Magnum and Magnum XL.

Putting on a condom the right way is very important. First, make sure it's not inside out. If you use a condom with a receptacle tip, gently press the air out of the tip before putting it on. Air bubbles can rupture condoms. If you use a condom with a plain tip, leave about an inch of space at the tip of the condom after pressing the air out; semen needs somewhere to go, and ejaculation without that space can cause a condom to break. Put a small amount of lube on the inside tip of the condom to reduce air bubbles and increase sensitivity.

If your partner has ejaculated during penetration, whether he feels his erection has subsided a little, all the way, or not at all, he should hold on to the base of the condom as he withdraws. By not holding on, he runs the risk of pulling out without the condom; then one of you has to fish around inside you for it, which is both awkward and unsafe, since semen could spill out of the condom. If he feels himself losing his erection during penetration or he withdraws before ejaculation, he should also hold on to the base.

There are dozens of brands and varieties of condoms on the market, and finding the right one for you may mean trying them out until you find one you love. The majority of condoms are made of latex, but people with latex allergies or sensitivities can try alternative materials like polyurethane from brands like Durex Avanti and Trojan Supra (only available with spermicide). Trojan Naturalambs, unique condoms made from lamb intestines, do not prevent STIs. These days, there are lots of styles to choose from: ribbed, studded, ridged, textured on the outside ("for her pleasure"), textured on the inside ("for his pleasure"), and many more.

Most condoms come prelubricated, but you can also buy unlubed condoms; either way, you can add your own favorite lube. You should never use a condom lubricated with nonoxynol-9. Nonoxynol-9, found in some lubricants and some lubricated condoms, is a chemical proven to kill the HIV virus and STIs in laboratory tests. Although it was once widely recommended for safer sex, we now know that many people are allergic to nonoxynol-9 and it really irritates their vaginas and rectums. Because nonoxynol-9 is so harsh on the delicate tissue of the vagina and rectum, research has shown that it's more likely to irritate or traumatize

Safer Sex Negotiation

Review each possible sexual/BDSM act and what your agreement is. Here are some questions to guide you:

Sex

- Hand jobs/external stimulation with hand: on penises, on vulvas
- External stimulation with a toy: on penises, on vulvas, on asses
- Oral sex: on penises, on vulvas, on asses
- Finger penetration: in vaginas, in asses
- Fisting: in vaginas, in asses
- Penetration with a toy: in vaginas, in asses
- Penetration with a penis: in vaginas, in asses

Within the categories, you should consider if there are particular rules about ejaculation and menstruation.

BDSM

- Genital play/"genitorture"
- Heavy impact play
- Play piercing
- Other kinds of play that may draw blood

the tissue, actually facilitating transmission of HIV and providing the virus with an accessible route to the bloodstream. Read condom labels to make sure the lube does not contain nonoxynol-9.

The Female Condom

The Reality Female Condom is a tube of polyurethane closed at one end and open at the other, like a larger version of the male condom. Although some women find them cumbersome, others say it gives them a sense of control and responsibility in the practice of safer sex. The female condom can be used for both vaginal and anal intercourse, and, in fact, it offers more protection because it lines the orifice, covering the penis and the outer area of the vulva or anus. The female condom can be slipped into the vagina or ass anytime before penetration. Before insertion, lubricate the outside of the condom, and make sure that the lubrication is evenly spread by rubbing the sides of the pouch together. To insert it, squeeze the sheath, and, starting with the inner ring, slip it in. Make sure that the inner ring is at the closed end of the pouch. Once it is inside, push it the rest of the way in with your finger. About an inch of the condom should hang outside the orifice, so the outer ring doesn't slip inside during the action.

During penetration, the condom may move around, either side to side or up and down. This is normal. However, if your partner's penis or dildo is long or thrusts deeply, the condom could slip all the way inside you. If your partner withdraws completely between thrusts, she or he could reenter outside the protection of the condom. If this happens, stop and adjust the condom. Like everything else, using the female condom takes practice and patience. To take the condom out, squeeze and twist the outer ring (to keep fluid inside the pouch) and pull it out slowly and gently. Don't flush the Reality Female Condom in the toilet—throw it away.

Making Sex Toys Safe

Transferring a sex toy from an infected person's vagina or anus directly to another person's vagina or anus puts the latter person at risk for STI transmission. You have a few options for making play with sex toys safe. Porous toys can be cleaned with soap and water or a sex toy cleaner, but cannot be completely disinfected. If a toy is porous (made of jelly, rubber, PVC, vinyl, or thermal plastic such as CyberSkin), you should either designate it as your own or, if you want to share it, cover it with a condom and change condoms when you change orifices or partners.

If a toy is made of a nonporous material like silicone, acrylic, glass, or metal, you can also cover it with a condom, or you can disinfect it before using it in a different orifice or with another partner. Silicone toys can be cleaned with hot water and antibacterial soap, a sex toy cleaner, or a diluted bleach solution (10:1 water-to-bleach); they can also be boiled for 5–10 minutes or put in the top rack of the dishwasher without detergent. Acrylic and glass toys can be cleaned with soap and water or the diluted bleach solution, and alcohol can be used on glass but not acrylic; always dry acrylic toys with a soft cloth, as paper towels can scratch them. For toys made of metal or other nonporous materials, follow the manufacturer's instructions for cleaning.

Sexually Transmitted Infections

All sexually active people should get medical checkups and genital exams (and for women, pelvic exams and Pap tests) on a regular basis. If you suspect you have an STI or you experience any unusual symptoms—bumps, rashes, sores, persistent itching, irritation, abdominal or pelvic pain, burning or pain during urination, any unusual discharge, irregular bleeding or cramping, or discomfort or pain during sex—you should see a doctor as soon as possible. *Many STIs may occur without any symptoms at all* and can only be detected through medical exams and laboratory tests. Most STIs can be treated and cured fairly easily with antibiotics or managed with other medications if they are caught in their early stages. Untreated STIs can lead to more serious complications, including sterility and cancer, so please take care of yourself. The information in this section should be used only as a guideline and is not a substitute for the advice of a doctor.

It is crucial that you find a health care professional you respect, trust, and feel comfortable talking to about your sexual health and practices. Many people feel embarrassed talking about health concerns, especially when it comes to their sexual health, but you need to be able to speak candidly about your symptoms and sexual practices to give your health care provider all the information needed to make a proper diagnosis.

In the discussion below about the transmission of STIs, I use the following terms for various forms of unprotected sex (sex without a safer sex barrier):

- *Rubbing:* manual external stimulation with fingers, without penetration, without a glove
- *Fingering:* vaginal or anal penetration with a finger or fingers, without a glove
- *Oral sex:* cunnilingus, fellatio, or analingus, without a barrier
- *Vaginal intercourse:* vaginal penetration with a penis, without a condom, with or without ejaculation
- *Anal intercourse:* anal penetration with a penis, without a condom, with or without ejaculation
- *Sharing sex toys:* transferring a sex toy from an infected person's orifice to another person's orifice without putting a condom on it or disinfecting it first

Chlamydia

Chlamydia is a sexually transmitted bacterial infection and the most common STI in the United States; it is estimated that there are 3 million cases every year. Chlamydia is found in semen, vaginal fluids, and secretions from the cervix. It can infect the vagina, urethra, cervix, anus, penis, eyes, or throat. It can be spread through vaginal and anal intercourse and oral sex, and more rarely from hand to eye, by sharing sex toys, or through rubbing and fingering if there are cuts in the skin.

Seventy-five percent of women and 50 percent of men with Chlamydia have no symptoms. If they do occur, symptoms can begin from five days to a few weeks after infection. In women, common symptoms include vaginal discharge, abdominal or stomach pain, painful penetration or urination, "breakthrough" menstrual bleeding (between periods), bowel movement discomfort, fever, swelling and soreness of the lymph nodes, and vaginal or rectal bleeding. Men may experience penile discharge, pain or burning during urination, and swelling and tenderness in the testicles or rectum. In cases of throat Chlamydia—most often passed to the partner who performs fellatio— you may develop a sore throat. Chlamydia is diagnosed by genital, pelvic, or rectal exam and treated with antibiotics such as doxycycline or azithromycin. If left untreated, Chlamydia can cause other serious problems, including pelvic inflammatory disease (PID) and infertility in men and women.[1]

Gonorrhea

Gonorrhea is a bacterial infection transmitted through various types of sexual contact, including vaginal and anal intercourse and oral sex, and less frequently by sharing sex toys and rubbing or fingering if there are cuts in the skin. Gonorrhea affects about 650,000 Americans every year. Approximately 75 percent of all reported cases are found in people aged 15 to 29. Gonorrhea is found in semen, vaginal fluids, and secretions from the cervix and can infect the vagina, urethra, cervix, anus, penis, or throat.

Up to 80 percent of women and about 10 percent of men who have gonorrhea have no symptoms; women are more likely to be asymptomatic in cases of rectal and throat gonorrhea than with vaginal gonorrhea. Symptoms appear within three to seven days of exposure and include, for men, penile discharge, pain or burning during urination, frequent urination, and rectal pain and discharge if gonorrhea is present in the rectum. Women may experience symptoms similar to those of Chlamydia: vaginal discharge, abdominal or stomach pain, vomiting, painful penetration or urination, "breakthrough" menstrual bleeding (between periods) or other irregularities with their period, fever, swelling and soreness of the vulva, and vaginal or rectal bleeding. Gonorrhea is diagnosed via a sample of urine, discharge, or cells from genital tissue and is treated with antibiotics, including penicillin, tetracycline, and ceftriaxone. Untreated gonorrhea can lead to ectopic pregnancy, pelvic inflammatory disease, and infertility in men and women.

Human Papillomavirus (HPV)

There are more than 100 types of the human papillomavirus (HPV), and more than 40 different strains can be sexually transmitted, affecting the vulva, vagina, cervix, penis, scrotum, anus, and rectum. Some strains of HPV are low risk, do not cause symptoms, and do not require treatment. Some strains cause genital warts, which are treatable. High-risk strains of HPV can cause abnormal cell growth, which may lead to cervical cancer in women and anal cancer in men and women.

According to Planned Parenthood, "At any time about 20 million people in the US have [genital HVP infections]. Between 10 and 15 million have high-risk types that are associated with cervical cancer. HPV is so common that about three out of four people have HPV at some point in their lives." The most common way to spread HPV is through vaginal and anal intercourse, but it can also be spread through rubbing, fingering, oral sex, or by sharing sex toys. Condoms protect against HPV, but because HPV may be present in skin that is not covered by a condom, gloves and dental dams should also be used.

When an HPV strain manifests as genital warts, warts can appear in as little as three weeks or as much as six months after infection. The warts begin as small pink bumps that look like tiny cauliflower florets in or around the genitals; they tend to spread rapidly, forming clumps that may be itchy or painful. Their incubation period is usually one to six months, but they can grow more rapidly if you are pregnant or have a compromised immune system. A person with HPV may have no external symptoms at all; in these cases, a physician will be able to see them during a genital, pelvic, or rectal exam. Some genital warts go away on their own. Or they can be removed by applying chemicals (usually acids), burning with an electric needle (electrocautery), freezing with liquid nitrogen (cryotherapy), or with laser treatment. Even after visible warts are removed, HPV remains in your body, and the warts can recur.

To test for high-risk strains of HPV that may cause precancerous or cancerous cells on the cervix, women can have a pelvic exam and a vaginal Pap smear (a swab of cells sent to a laboratory for analysis). The Pap test can detect abnormal cell changes; if the Pap results come back abnormal, the woman should have the cells tested specifically for the HPV virus. If the HPV virus is detected, doctors often perform a colposcopy to get a closer look at the cells before deciding on a treatment plan.

Men who contract HPV may develop genital warts or show no symptoms, remaining carriers of the virus who can pass it on to their partners. Men can be tested for HPV with a penile cell smear. At least one strain of HPV has been linked to cancer of the penis, which is very rare in the United States.

HPV is much more likely to cause precancerous or cancerous cells in the cervix than in the rectum; however, HPV can also occur in the rectums of both men and women and can lead to anal cancer. Men and women can be tested for rectal HPV with a rectal exam and an anal Pap smear. HPV can be spread from a woman's ass to her vagina, and vice versa, so if it has been discovered in one place, you're advised to get the other orifice checked.

Persons diagnosed with a high-risk strain of HPV should get regular exams to monitor recurrences and prevent complications. Depending on the strain, the part of the body where HPV is found, and the severity of cellular changes, precancerous cells may be removed by cryotherapy, laser treatment, or a loop electrosurgical excision procedure (LEEP).[2]

In 2006, a vaccine for girls and women was released that can prevent four strains of HPV: two strains account for 90 percent of cases of genital warts and two account for 70 percent of cervical cancer cases. The vaccine, currently marketed under the name Gardasil, is recommended by the FDA for girls and women aged 9–26. However, women over 26 who have not been exposed to all strains of HPV can also benefit from the vaccine. Several drug companies are conducting clinical trials on the vaccination of boys and men.

Genital Herpes

Herpes simplex virus type 1 (HSV-1) is the virus that usually causes oral herpes, found in an estimated 50–80 percent of the US population. According to Planned Parenthood, about 25 percent of American adults have herpes simplex virus type 2 (HSV-2), the virus that usually causes genital herpes. Genital herpes is transmitted through sexual contact, including vaginal and anal intercourse and oral sex, and, less commonly, rubbing or fingering with cuts in the skin and sharing sex toys. The virus can be transmitted by skin-to-skin contact if one person is currently having an outbreak or during a period known as "asymptomatic shedding," when the person has no symptoms but is still infectious. Condoms and dental dams can help reduce the risk; however, if a sore is present on a part of the body not covered by the condom or dam, the virus can still be spread.

When a person first contracts genital herpes, there may be few or no noticeable symptoms. If symptoms develop (usually within 2–20 days after infection, but as late as several years afterward), the initial outbreak is often worse than subsequent outbreaks. The person may experience a tingly or burning sensation in the genital area; then bumps, blisters, or open sores appear in the affected area, which can be itchy, sore, or painful. Women may experience flulike symptoms, swollen glands or lymph nodes, a vaginal discharge or yeast infection, and painful urination. Initial sores usually heal in one to three weeks without treatment.

Once you become infected with the herpes virus, you have the antibodies in your system and cannot be reinfected in the part of your body where you were previously infected; however, though it's much less common after the initial outbreak, you can be infected in other areas. So, if you've only had outbreaks in or around your vagina, you can still spread genital herpes to other parts of your body by having unprotected sex with another herpes carrier.

Herpes is a chronic infection, and symptoms can recur during outbreaks. These outbreaks can be brought on by stress, a compromised immune system, or prolonged exposure to the sun; they can last for up to three weeks. During an outbreak, most experts recommend that you refrain from oral sex and intercourse, even with a barrier. Although a person is most contagious during an outbreak, transmission of the virus can occur during inactive periods as well (especially during the two weeks after an outbreak), with or without visible blisters or other symptoms. Doctors prescribe medications such as acyclovir, famiciclovir, or valacyclovir to both treat and prevent outbreaks, but there is no cure for genital herpes.[3]

People who have multiple sex partners must be aware of certain daunting aspects of genital herpes. If you have a cold sore caused by type 1 herpes and perform cunnilingus on your partner, she can develop type 2 genital herpes.[4] People with herpes can be symptom-free for quite some time, believing they are free of the virus, yet still pass it on to others. People with herpes often assume that they're not contagious if they aren't having an outbreak, but they are actually contagious. If a potential partner is symptom-free, you have no way of knowing they have genital herpes unless they tell you. Even if you always use condoms, you can still give genital herpes to someone or get it from them.

Syphilis

In the US fewer than 40,000 cases of syphilis are reported each year. Syphilis is a bacterial infection that is transmitted by touching a sore on an infected person; sores can appear on the mouth, penis, vagina, anus, or skin. You can spread it through vaginal and anal intercourse, oral sex, rubbing or fingering (especially but not exclusively if there are cuts in the skin) and very rarely, by sharing sex toys.

Syphilis has an incubation period of two to eight weeks. Ten to 90 days after exposure, infected persons experience the primary stage of the virus. A round ulcer (called a chancre) erupts in the affected area, usually where the bacteria entered the body; common locations are the vulva, labia, foreskin, scrotum, or the base of the penis. Sores may also appear on the cervix, tongue, lips, and other areas. The chancre and surrounding area may ache or burn—or not. The infected person may have swollen lymph nodes.

After the chancre hardens, heals, and disappears, the secondary stage begins. This stage is marked by a general skin rash, with sores the size of pennies that may be itchy and painful. You may experience fever, swollen glands, aching joints, headaches, nausea, and constipation. People are most contagious during the secondary stage. The third and fourth stages, which are latent stages of tertiary syphilis, are very serious and can be deadly if untreated. Syphilis is diagnosed by blood testing and testing fluid from the sores. People who have had syphilis for less than a year can be treated with antibiotics, usually penicillin, doxycycline, or tetracycline.

Hepatitis A

Five types of hepatitis, an inflammatory liver disease, have been identified: A through E. The most common are hepatitis A, B, and C. The
hepatitis A virus (HAV) is transmitted when infected fecal matter gets
into the bloodstream, usually by ingesting contaminated food. *If you
practice unprotected oral-anal sex with an infected person and come into
contact with their fecal matter, you are at risk.* There are conflicting studies about how many cases of HAV are spread through sexual contact.

On average, the incubation period is 30 days, but it can range from
14 to 60 days. An individual is most infectious two weeks before and
one week after he or she develops symptoms. Symptoms include
fatigue, nausea, vomiting, abdominal pain, dark urine, light stools,
fever, and jaundice (yellowing of the skin and eyes). You may become
ill with several of these symptoms suddenly. Doctors can diagnose hepatitis A with a blood test. There is no treatment for hepatitis A, and
it usually clears up on its own in weeks or months, depending on a
person's immune system; the liver repairs itself and there is no perma-
nent damage. Once you've had it, you develop antibodies for it and
cannot become ill with it again. In the United States, nearly 100,000
new cases of HAV are reported every year. There is a vaccine for the
virus.[5]

Hepatitis B

The type of hepatitis most likely to be sexually transmitted is hepatitis
B, caused by the hepatitis B virus (HBV). The virus is present in all
bodily fluids of an infected person, including semen, saliva, vaginal
secretions, blood, feces, menstrual blood, and sweat, though it can
only be transmitted through blood, semen, and possibly saliva. It can
be spread through vaginal and anal intercourse and analingus, and
through manual penetration if there is a cut on the skin and a tear in
rectal tissue or rectal bleeding. *HBV is 100 times easier to transmit sexually than HIV.* About 80,000 Americans become infected with HBV

each year. One out of 20 people in the United States will become infected with HBV sometime during their lives. Most of these infections occur among people 20 to 49 years old. There is an HBV vaccine to prevent hepatitis B; it is given in multiple scheduled doses over four to six months.

About 50 percent of adults with HBV never develop symptoms. When symptoms do occur, they appear between six weeks and six months after infection and may mimic flu symptoms: fatigue, nausea, vomiting, loss of appetite, headache, fever, tenderness and pain in the lower abdomen or joints, and possibly jaundice; more severe symptoms include hives, severe abdominal pain, dark urine, and light stools. Hepatitis B is diagnosed by a blood test.

About 95 percent of adults who contract hepatitis B acquire the acute form of the disease; they develop antibodies to the virus and recover within two to six months without medication or treatment. While their blood will always test positive to the virus, they are immune and are not infectious. The other 5 percent become chronically infected. They may or may not continue to show symptoms, but they will always be a carrier of the virus and can infect other people; they are at risk of developing cirrhosis, liver failure, and liver cancer. There are about 1.25 million HBV carriers in the United States. While there is no treatment or cure for acute hepatitis B, people with chronic hepatitis are prescribed various medications to eradicate or suppress the replication of the virus.[6]

Hepatitis C

Hepatitis C, caused by the hepatitis C virus (HCV), is passed from person to person through direct contact with an infected person's blood. It is primarily spread through unsafe IV drug use, including sharing needles. Researchers disagree on the number of cases transmitted through sexual contact. Some studies "failed to detect the presence of HCV in either saliva, semen, or urine of HCV-infected people—

except when those body fluids have been contaminated by the person's blood."[7] Other sources state that it is present in blood, semen, and vaginal fluids, but that semen and vaginal fluids are much less effective at transmitting the virus.[8] It may be spread through vaginal and anal intercourse, but only when there are tears in the tissue or bleeding, and through finger-fucking with bleeding *and* cuts on the skin of the finger. HCV is more likely to be spread during sex if one partner also has HIV or another sexually transmitted infection.

Most infected people are asymptomatic or show mild symptoms that resemble the flu: nausea, fatigue, loss of appetite, fever, headaches, and abdominal pain. HCV is diagnosed by a blood test. Twenty to 30 percent of infected persons can become disease-free with medication that contains the viral activity and reproduction and decreases inflammation in the liver. A large percentage, about 70–80 percent, contract chronic hepatitis C, and many of this group develop cirrhosis (scarring of the liver) or liver failure. Hepatitis C can be fatal in some cases. There is no vaccine for HCV.[9]

HIV and AIDS

HIV, the virus that causes AIDS, is transmitted through bodily fluids and is most concentrated in blood and semen, and present in menstrual blood, breast milk, and vaginal secretions. HIV is transmitted in several ways: through unprotected sexual contact with the bodily fluids of an infected person, by sharing needles with an infected person (engaging in intravenous drug use), by receiving infected blood (through a transfusion), or from mother to baby via amniotic fluid during delivery or breast-feeding.

Each year in the United States there are about 40,000 new cases of HIV/AIDS; 930,000 cases of AIDS have been reported to the Centers for Disease Control and Prevention to date. Some people develop symptoms soon after they are infected, but it can take up to 10 years to become symptomatic. Early symptoms include headaches, fever, diarrhea, muscle pain, weakness, fatigue, night sweats, and swollen glands. A patient in the later stage of the disease may experience a wide range of more serious symptoms that differ depending on the person.

It's easier for women to get HIV from men through vaginal intercourse than vice versa. The tissue of the vagina is more susceptible than the tissue of the penis to trauma, tears, and minute sores, which provide infected precum and semen a direct route to the bloodstream. During anal intercourse, it's easier for the receptive partner to get HIV from the insertive partner for similar reasons: the tissue of the rectum is even more delicate than that of the vagina. In addition, the viral load of HIV is higher in semen than in vaginal fluids, so infected semen is more infectious than infected vaginal secretions. Both women and men can also get the virus, much less commonly, through oral sex, and possibly through sharing toys and rubbing and fingering if there are cuts on the skin and in vaginal or rectal tissue.

AIDS can be diagnosed through oral swab, urine, and blood tests. The most common tests detect the antibodies for HIV, not the HIV virus itself. In most cases, antibodies appear in the body within four weeks; however, it can take up to three months for an infected person to develop antibodies. A more expensive test, the PCR-DNA test, tests for the HIV virus itself, detecting its presence in the blood within three to seven days of exposure. However, it is not currently approved by the Food and Drug Administration (FDA). An infected person can infect others between the time of infection and the detection of antibodies or virus.[10]

There is no cure for AIDS, but there have been many advances in the treatment of the disease. For many, HIV has become a manageable chronic illness. With various combinations of prescription medications, people with HIV and AIDS are living longer, healthier lives now than in the past.

Chapter 19

Legal and Practical Issues

THE INSTITUTIONS OF MAINSTREAM SOCIETY, including the law, conspicuously fail to acknowledge or support people in nontraditional relationships. People in polyamorous relationships are often unable to marry the partner of their choice to legally protect their relationships and share in certain benefits. They may marry or register as domestic partners with one of their partners, leaving other partners out in the cold, legally speaking. Whether you are a polyamorous person with three partners, one member of a committed quad, or living with your chosen family, you should know what your options are for protecting yourself, your loved ones, and your assets. Laws, policies, and procedures that affect everyday life as well as critically important life decisions are not set up for unconventional relationships—you must educate yourself and be creative. This is a brief overview of some of the practical and legal issues people in nonmonogamous relationships face.

Housing Laws

Federal Fair Housing Acts prohibits housing discrimination on the basis of race, religion, national origin, gender, age, familial status (whether you have children), and physical or mental disability. These federal laws do not protect people based on their marital status. A landlord can ask about your marital status and choose not to rent to you based on the fact that you are unmarried or in some form of alternative relationship. A few states have legislation on the books that bans discrimination based on marital status, but the language often refers to unmarried couples—not an unmarried triad, for example. When applying to rent, it's probably safer not to out yourselves. If you're in a triad, you could tell a potential landlord you are a couple with a roommate, or three friends. Leases usually specify the maximum number of occupants, so make sure to read the fine print carefully before you sign one.

Property Ownership

When two or more persons jointly purchase real estate, there are several options for how to structure ownership. If you purchase the property together, the structure you choose will be recorded on the property title. If one partner owns property and you want to add additional partners to the title, you should consult a lawyer about legal issues and procedures and an accountant about possible tax implications.

Joint Tenancy

In joint tenancy, also referred to as joint tenancy with rights of survivorship, each person owns an equal share of the property. When one tenant dies, his share goes to the surviving tenants. The main benefit of joint tenancy is that property shares are distributed to the surviving owners without having to go through probate court, which can be expensive and time-consuming. Some states have specific guidelines for joint tenancy, and others limit the number of parties to joint tenancy with rights of survivorship, so make sure to research the laws in your area and check with a legal advisor.

Tenancy in Common

There is no limit to the number of people who can hold the title of a property as tenants in common. And tenants in common do not have to hold equal shares of the property; it can be divided however the owners want. When one owner dies, his share of the property goes to whomever he specifies in his will or trust. Unlike joint tenancy, property owned by tenants in common must go through probate court. If you or another partner want to leave your share of the property to children or other heirs, this may be a better option for you. You might also consider tenancy in common with life estate provision: upon your death, the other owners can remain in the property until they die, whereupon all shares are passed to the designated heirs.

Zoning Laws and Enforceable Rules

Some towns, counties, and cities have zoning laws that limit the number of adults unrelated biologically or by marriage who can live in a single-family residence. This means your dream of a five-person poly collective in that big Victorian house may actually be against the law or in violation of a housing ordinance. Especially when purchasing property, make sure you educate yourself in the local zoning laws and read the fine print in a property's deed restrictions. If the property is part of a subdivision, community, or other entity with a governing body (such as a homeowners' association, condo board, or co-op board), investigate the rules before you sign on the dotted line.

Employment Benefits

Health Insurance

All health insurance companies recognize and provide coverage for married couples, and some now extend coverage to domestic partners as well, provided you are registered in your city, county, or state. In some cases, a state may not recognize domestic partnerships, but an employer recognizes them for the purposes of spousal benefits. Talk to your employer about their particular policies and eligibility requirements. No health insurance company extends benefits to more than one partner or spouse of an employee.

Life Insurance, Retirement Accounts, Pensions

Most life insurance companies permit co-beneficiaries or multiple beneficiaries to receive the proceeds of a life insurance policy. The same is true for retirement accounts and pensions. Alternatively, you may designate a trust as the beneficiary and, through a will, name multiple partners to share in the trust. If you don't have a will, these benefits go to your next of kin.

Creating a Corporation

Some people in polyfidelitous relationships have opted to form a business to protect certain assets of their relationships. There are various kinds of corporations, and laws vary by state, but creating a corporation may be a good option for sharing finances and ownership of assets and for obtaining health insurance and other benefits. For example, you can split the ownership of substantial property, like a house, into percentages so each person owns a specified number of shares in the corporation. Creating and running a corporation involves maintaining records, filing lots of documentation with the state, paying corporate taxes, and other administrative work which may or may not outweigh the benefits.

Legal Designations and Documents

Durable Power of Attorney

A Durable Power of Attorney is a legal document in which you designate one or more persons ("agents") to make financial, medical, health care, and other decisions for you if you're unable to make them yourself. The financial matters your designated agent is empowered to take charge of include: handling financial transactions, managing bank accounts, paying bills, collecting money owed to you, and investing your money; filing and paying taxes; buying, selling, and maintaining real estate; and signing legal documents on your behalf. You may designate one person to oversee these areas as well as make medical decisions (outlined below), or designate one person for financial matters (via a Durable Power of Attorney for Finances) and another for health-care matters. You may appoint multiple agents to act on your behalf; however, if you do, you must spell out whether each agent can act separately or if they must all make decisions together.

Health Care Proxy/Durable Medical Power of Attorney

Use a health care proxy, also called a Durable Medical or Health Care Power of Attorney, to designate who will make medical decisions on your behalf should you be unable to do so; the designated person is called an agent or proxy. If you become unconscious, unable to communicate, mentally incapacitated, or in some way not competent to make decisions, your health care proxy or proxies will be empowered to make important decisions about your health care (including medical treatments and whether to provide or remove life-sustaining treatment, as well as who can visit you in the hospital).

If no health care proxy or durable medical power of attorney exists, your next of kin is empowered to make decisions about your medical care and who can visit you. Hospitals and medical facilities have differing policies, but some allow visitation only by next of kin and "immediate family" (meaning biological relatives). Today, more health-care institutions have policies that allow same-sex, domestic, and unmarried partners to visit each other and participate in decision making. However, these are policies not laws; they are implemented at the discretion of hospital administrators, who may or may not be supportive of your alternative family. You may also sign a Hospital Visitation Directive to specify individuals (related to you or not) whom you do or do not want to visit you in the hospital. Each state has slightly different laws stipulating what decisions a health care proxy can make, so it's important to get legal advice. You may appoint multiple agents, but if you do, you must spell out whether each agent can act separately or if they must all make decisions together.

Living Will

Most people who appoint a medical proxy also draw up a living will, a document that outlines what types of medical treatments and life support you want at the end of your life. This is an important document that expresses your wishes concerning these life-or-death decisions and guides your health care proxy in making them.

Will

If you die without a will, everything in your estate—including life insurance, bank accounts, investments, property—will be left to your next of kin, defined by the courts as your legal spouse or your closest living blood relative. By drawing up a will, you can designate who will manage your estate and to whom your assets will be distributed.

Disposition of Remains

Disposition of Remains is the legal term for what happens to your body after you die. Oddly, your body does not belong to your estate, as you might assume. You must designate someone to be in charge of it; otherwise, it is turned over to your next of kin. If you have particular wishes regarding burial or cremation, or where you want to be buried or have your ashes spread, you should specify who will be in charge of your remains.

Children

Attorney Valerie White recommends that multiple partners who want to raise children together engage in thoughtful planning and consideration. Before a child is born, she says, all the parents should sit down and write an agreement stating their intentions with regard to custody, visitation, and support in case the relationship breaks up. You may want to consult a lawyer or other advisor when creating this document.

Parentage

"Say there are two men and one woman in a triad. The woman becomes pregnant, and the three agree that they don't care who the biological father of the baby is, since they all consider themselves parents. They have the romantic notion that they don't want to know and don't need to know," White says. "There are still lots of good reasons—inheritance, child support, medical issues—to know who the biological father is."[1] White recommends that if you and your partners absolutely don't want to know the paternity, you should have the DNA testing done and place the sealed results in a safe place, so that the child can access the information when needed.

Legal Guardianship

The known biological parents of a child are listed on the child's birth certificate, and the state considers them the legal parents. If an adult who is not related to a child wants to become her parent (for example, gay and lesbian parents, stepparents), the adult may adopt the child. However, no more than two adults can adopt a child, making adoption not an option for polyamorous and polyfidelitous partners. In a triad, for example, two partners who are the biological parents may want the other partner to have custody of the child, equal parental rights, and the legal right to make medical and other important decisions. In certain states, you may petition the family court to become a co-guardian of the child. In most cases—usually where the legal guardians are incapacitated, incompetent, or die suddenly—someone petitions to be a co-guardian *instead* of the legal guardians. In this case, you want to be a co-guardian *in addition to* the legal guardians. Procedures differ in each state and include filing a petition, meeting with a social worker, and testifying before a judge. Valerie White did this with her two triad partners: "We told them we were an intentional family of three." It's rare for a judge to reject an agreement agreed to by both legal parents.

Custody Disputes

When it comes to disputes over custody, unfortunately, there is no legal precedent or strong legal support for alternative families, including gay and lesbian families and polyamorous ones. In fact it's quite the opposite: in many custody cases people's open relationships have been used against them.

Cat, a 38-year-old massage therapist who lives in Oklahoma, lost custody of her children in part because of her polyamory. She and her ex-husband were married for 11 years and polyamorous beginning in the second year. Ten years down the road, he met a woman at work, they fell in love, and four months later he left Cat. "Then he went completely opposite of everything we had done: he went to monogamy and Christianity," Cat says. He used what was once also his lifestyle against her in court. "He basically spent five years trying to win custody of the kids, and then finally in the last year [he did]. It was based somewhat on my political activity because I'm a pretty outspoken political radical here. But also the killing points in my custody case were my open relationships, my relationships with queer people and trans people, and my willingness to be open and not hide my lifestyle. In Oklahoma, it was just damning."

Valerie White says, "It's all too frequent, tragic, and sad that a former spouse decides to sue for custody because he or she believes that it is just not okay for the kid to live with the polyamorous parent.

Other Issues to Consider

Property titles: Some forms of property cannot be titled to more than two people. For example, in some states, the Department of Motor Vehicles cannot issue a title for a car in the name of more than two people—even if there is proof that more than two people purchased it. In some cases, it's simply because the computer system is designed to accept a maximum of two names.

Parole and probation: If you are on parole or probation, in many jurisdictions you must agree "to lead an exemplary life," where "exemplary" is not specifically defined. Parole and probation officers, who have a great deal of leeway and power in these matters, can decide that your having multiple partners is a violation of this condition.

Employment contracts: Many employers require that new employees sign an employment contract when they're hired. Some of these agreements contain a so-called morals clause, which your relationship style may violate. A morals clause usually includes wording such as "The employee shall conduct himself with due regard to public convention and morals." While there are no known cases of someone being fired for being polyamorous, it is possible and absolutely legal.

Emigration and immigration: A man with multiple wives who is immigrating to the United States from a country where polygamy is legal cannot legally bring all his wives with him, because the US bans the practice of polygamy. Likewise, if you live in a poly relationship in the US and one spouse gets a job in Canada, he or she can emigrate with the legal spouse and children, but not with other partners or nonlegal spouses.

Sometimes, one parent decides that he or she wants custody and uses the other parent's lifestyle as a club. Too often people are threatened with loss of custody." Even if poly parents create an agreement that covers issues like custody, visitation, and support, White warns, "What the court sees as the 'best interests of the child' can trump anything that the parents have agreed to."

Chapter 20

The Future of Relationships

WHEN THE NEWS BROKE IN 1998 that President Bill Clinton had had a sexual affair with Monica Lewinsky, some people speculated that he and his wife, Hillary, had "an agreement." There was proof that Bill had been sleeping with other women for most of their marriage, and talk that Hillary not only knew about it, but tolerated the affairs (a theory that was posited again in several books about the Clintons published later). Neither one has ever admitted to having any sort of consensual pact. Some who believe they did used that notion to paint Hillary as a calculating, power-hungry politician. I was just fascinated that Americans could be standing around the water cooler considering whether the President and the First Lady had a deal, an understanding—an open relationship. Whether they did or they still do, the public will never know. But the notion that it is even a possibility represents just how much society's ideas about marriage and monogamy have changed.

Much of the credit for this change must be given to the women's movement and the GLBT civil rights movement. Feminists and queer people have been instrumental in challenging "either/or" standards, gender roles, sexuality taboos, and relationship models. They have also redefined what it means to be a family. In late 2003, nonmonogamy again became a public talking point when the debate over gay marriage dominated the political landscape. Those in favor of gay marriage fought to challenge heterosexism and redefine commitment and matrimony. Opponents used the issue to strike fear into the hearts of Americans by linking sanctioned queer coupling with other kinds of relationships—the polyamorous and the preposterous. The argument went something like this: *If we allow gay people to get married, what will be next? Three people getting hitched? Someone marrying their dog? It's a slippery slope.* Unfortunately, some gay activists took the bait and vehemently denounced other kinds of alternative relationships.

It's ironic that polyamorous people found themselves left at the altar by some queers. Both groups are fighting for the same thing: the recognition of relationships that contradict the dominant model—heterosexual and monogamous. It remains to be seen where the gay marriage debate will land and what impact it will have for everyone who isn't "straight" in one way or another. While polyamorous people have become organized, they—along with others in open relationships—must mobilize, pick up the baton, and run even farther with it. We have accepted that Heather has two mommies; now it's time to acknowledge that Heather's mommies may have secondary partners, lovers, or friends with benefits.

In *The Future of Love*, Daphne Rose Kingma writes: "Our whole world of relationships is in an uproar… It's as if we awoke one morning to discover that a blizzard of transformation occurred during the night."[1] Public discussion—spurred by the Clinton sex scandal, the gay marriage debate, and even HBO's new show about polygamists, *Big Love*—demonstrates that nonmonogamy is making its way into the mainstream discourse. The blizzard of transformation continues unabated.

Further proof of this transformation is the 126 people I interviewed for this book, a fraction of the much larger population who are in consensual nonmonogamous relationships and marriages all over the United States. They are living examples of a shift in the way we do relationships.

Their stories represent the amazing diversity of the people who choose some form of nonmonogamy and the ways they design their open relationships. In a society where people feel isolated and dissatisfied with monogamy, where cheating and dishonesty are rampant, nonmonogamous relationships reflect a new strategy—one that is honest and brave, that strives to bring people together through multipartner relationships, networks, and communities.

It's no coincidence that many of the people who are living in open relationships have defied societal norms in other ways. Confronted with binary choices such as gay or straight, male or female, husband or wife, they literally or figuratively choose "other" as they attempt to expand the definitions. Faced with the cultural dichotomies of friend/lover, single/married, casual/committed, and faithful/unfaithful, they refuse to conform. Their courage to be fluid and defy categories is a beacon of how relationships will continue to change in the 21st century. Let them inspire you to redefine your relationship(s) on your terms.

I hope *Opening Up* has given you a look at the inner workings of modern relationships as well as tools and strategies you can employ in the care and feeding of your open relationship. I conclude with words of advice from the folks I interviewed about what it takes to create and sustain open relationships.

Anything valuable worth holding on to requires a lot of hard work and some difficult moments. —David

Take it slow, stay patient, be persistent, be willing to listen to everyone's emotions. Remember, it's all about love. —Marissa

It's so important for people to feel that they have freedom to choose what works best for them instead of having to fall into somebody else's prescribed pattern. —Cat

Poly has been, for me, a lot about letting go. Letting go of fear, of expectations, of self-imposed limitations. —Barbara

If you're trying to do the right thing in life and by the people you love and who love you, then you're already ahead of the game.
—Kathleen

I have faith in my primary partner's love. For as long as we remain confident of each other's essential loyalty and commitment, we don't suffer anxiety over the possibility of losing what we have together. —Eli

Truly evaluating yourself and knowing yourself, seeing your flaws and strengths as objectively as you can muster, will help you understand how to relate to someone else—even multiple people. That keen self-awareness can inform you of why you make the choices you do, what patterns have been holding you back, when you were at your happiest, and why. You can do so much for yourself by just being honest about your mistakes and triumphs—and once you do, sharing that with someone else is easy and fulfilling.
—Bella

Let your relationships be what they are. Relationships seem to have their own trajectories, their own needs and wants and expiration dates, their own purposes. Being open to how relationships grow and shift is very difficult and very necessary. Sometimes a friend becomes a lover, a lover becomes a friend, sometimes the right person appears at exactly the right time for a specific purpose. (And then, when that purpose is done, sometimes disappears entirely. Cancer victims often experience this with their "cancer buddies.") Sometimes the perfect relationship to have with someone is an extravagant dinner and delicious sex—twice a year. Even if they live around the corner. —Bear

The most fundamental element is a desire for growth for you and your partner. —Juan

Once you leave the beaten path of a traditional monogamous relationship, you really are off in the forest where anything is possible. You are only limited by your imagination. —Owen

Notes

Introduction

1. David P. Barash and Judith Eve Lipton, *The Myth of Monogamy: Fidelity and Infidelity in Animals and People* (Henry Holt, 2001), 149.

2. Philip Blumstein and Pepper Schwartz, *American Couples: Money, Work, Sex* (William Morrow, 1983), 30.

3. Ibid.

4. US Census Bureau statistics quoted in Barbara Dafoe Whitehead and David Popenoe, "Social Indicators Of Marital Health and Well-being: Trends of the Past Four Decades," *The State of Our Unions: The Social Health of Marriage in America 2005*, http://marriage. rutgers.edu/Publications/SOOU/TEXTSOOU2005.htm.

5. In 1960, the rate was 73.5 per 1,000 unmarried women age 15 and older; in 2004, the rate was 39.9 per 1,000 unmarried women age 15 and older. The difference is 45.71 percent. US Census Bureau statistics quoted in Whitehead and Popenoe, "Social Indicators of Marital Health and Well-being."

6. Joshua R. Goldstein, "The Leveling of Divorce in the United States," *Demography* 36 (1999): 409–414; Andrew Cherlin, *Marriage, Divorce, Remarriage* (Cambridge, Mass.: Harvard University Press, 1992), cited in David Popenoe, "The Top Ten Myths of Divorce," http://marriage.rutgers.edu/Publications/pubtoptenmyths.htm.

7. Samuel S. Janus and Cynthia L. Janus, *The Janus Report on Sexual Behavior* (Wiley, 1993), 169, 196. The data reported in the 1993 book was based on research conducted from 1988 to 1992.

8. Jane Weaver, "Many Cheat for a Thrill, More Stay True for Love," *Today*, April 16, 2007, http://today.msnbc.msn.com/id/17951664.

9. I want to acknowledge that I am a part of the media's obsession with relationship dissatisfaction and I have benefited from that dissatisfaction in some ways. I have taught workshops on improving sex life, and my sex books are part of the large self-help section in bookstores.

10. George Bernard Shaw, *Man and Superman*, quoted at http://www notable-quotes.com/s/shaw_george_bernard.html.

Chapter 1

1. Terry Gould, *The Lifestyle: A Look at the Erotic Rites of Swingers* (Firefly Books, 2000); Liberated Christians, http://www.libchrist.com/swing/began.html; Wikipedia entry on swinging, http://en.wiki pedia.org/wiki/Swinging; Curtis Bergstrand and Jennifer Blevins Williams, "Today's Alternative Marriage Styles: The Case of Swingers," Electronic Journal of Human Sexuality, Vol. 3, October 10, 2000, http://www.ejhs.org/volume3/swing/body.htm.

2. William Breedlove and Jerrye Breedlove, *Swap Clubs: A Study in Contemporary Sexual Mores* (Sherbourne Press, 1964).

3. "The History," Lifestyles Forum, April 9, 2007, http://www.lifestylesforum.com/www/wp/?p=7.

4. Gould, *The Lifestyle*, 76.

5. Carolyn Symonds, "Sexual Mate Swapping: Violation of Norms and Reconciliation of Guilt," in *Studies in the Sociology of Sex*, James M. Henslin, ed. (Appleton-Century-Crofts, 1971), 82–83.

6. Nena O'Neill and George O'Neill, "Open Marriage: The Conceptual Framework," in *Beyond Monogamy: Recent Studies of Sexual Alternatives in Marriage*, James R. Smith and Lynn G. Smith, eds. (Johns Hopkins University Press, 1974), 62.

7. Larry L. Constantine and Joan M. Constantine, *Group Marriage: A Study of Contemporary Multilateral Marriage* (Macmillan, 1973), 28–29.

8. Allan Bérubé, "The History of Gay Bathhouses," in *Policing Public Sex: Queer Politics and the Future of AIDS Activism*, Dangerous Bedfellows, ed. (Boston: South End Press, 1996), 188.

9. Ibid., 187–220.

10. Gayle Rubin, "The Catacombs: A Temple of the Butthole," in *Leatherfolk: Radical Sex, People, Politics, and Practice*, Mark Thompson, ed. (Alyson Publications, 1991), 139.

11. Jack Fritscher, "The Catacombs: Fistfucking in a Handball Palace," *Drummer* 23, July 1978, http://www.jackfritscher.com/Drummer/Articles/Catacombs.html.

12. Thyme S. Siegel, "Matriarchal Village," in *The Lesbian Polyamory Reader: Open Relationships, Non-Monogamy, and Casual Sex*, Marcia Munson and Judith P. Stelboum, eds. (Binghamton, N.Y.: Haworth Press, 1999), 127.

13. Kerista website, http://www.kerista.com/herstory.html.

14. Ryam Nearing and Taj Anapol, "Polyamory: A Personal and Historical Retrospective," *Loving More* no. 32, Winter 2003, 12–15.

15. The Ravenhearts, "Frequently Asked Questions Re: Polyamory," http://www.mithrilstar.org/Polyamory-FAQ-Ravenhearts.htm.

16. Philip Blumstein and Pepper Schwartz, *American Couples: Money, Work, Sex* (William and Morrow, 1983), 312.

17. Samuel S. Janus and Cynthia L. Janus, *The Janus Report on Sexual Behavior* (Wiley, 1993), 184. The data reported in the 1993 book was based on research conducted from 1988 to 1992.

18. E. H. Page, "Mental Health Services Experiences of Bisexual Women and Bisexual Men: An Empirical Study," *Journal of Bisexuality* vol. 3, issue 3/4 (2004): 137–160, cited in Geri Weitzman, "Therapy with Clients Who Are Bisexual and Polyamorous," *Journal of Bisexuality* vol. 6, issue 1/2 (2006): 137–164.

19. The number of people who responded to the survey was cited on *The Oprah Winfrey Show*, episode no 8641, "237 Reasons to Have Sex," September 25, 2007 (Harpo Productions; ABC). The percentage was reported on the Oprah.com website, http://www2.oprah.com/relationships/sex/relationships_sex_284_112.jhtml.

Chapter 2

1. David P. Barash and Judith Eve Lipton, *The Myth of Monogamy: Fidelity and Infidelity in Animals and People* (Henry Holt, 2001), 1.

2. Ibid., 11.

3. Brooke Adams, "Fundamentalists: Most Espouse Polygamy as a Tenet, but Fewer Actually Practice It as Their Lifestyle," *Salt Lake Tribune*, August 11, 2005.

4. S. A. Peabody, "Alternative Life Styles to Monogamous Marriage: Variants of Normal Behavior in Psychotherapy Clients," *Family Relations* 31 (1982): 425–434, and A. M. Rubin, "Sexually Open Versus Sexually Exclusive Marriage: A Comparison of Dyadic Adjustment," *Alternative Lifestyles* 5 (1982): 101–106, cited in Geri D. Weitzman, "What Psychology Professionals Should Know About Polyamory," www.polyamory.org/~joe/polypaper.htm, March 1999.

5. Peabody, "Alternative Life Styles to Monogamous Marriage," cited in Weitzman, "What Psychology Professionals Should Know About Polyamory."

Chapter 3

1. Steve Curwood, "The Chemistry of Love," interview with Helen Fisher, February 3, 2006, http://www.loe.org/shows/segments.htm?programID=06-P13–00005&segmentID=7.
2. John Caldwell, "Gay Men, Straight Lives," *Advocate*, October 12, 2004.
3. Amity Pierce Buxton, *The Other Side of the Closet: The Coming-Out Crisis for Straight Spouses and Families* (Wiley, 1994), cited in Caldwell, "Gay Men, Straight Lives."
4. Buxton, "Works in Progress: How Mixed-Orientation Couples Maintain their Marriages after the Wives Come Out," *Journal of Bisexuality* vol. 4, no. 1/2 (2004): 79.

Chapter 4

1. Personal interview with Anita Wagner, August 6, 2007.
2. PuddleDancer Press website, http://www.nonviolentcommunication.com/aboutnvc/aboutnvc.htm.
3. Marshall B. Rosenberg, *Nonviolent Communication: A Language of Life*, 2nd ed. (Encinitas, Calif.: PuddleDancer Press, 2003).
4. Brad Blanton, *Radical Honesty: How to Transform Your Life by Telling the Truth* (Stanley, Va.: Sparrowhawk Publications, 2003), 63.
5. Personal interview with Mark Michaels and Patricia Johnson, July 27, 2007.
6. Ibid.
7. Ronald Mazur, *The New Intimacy: Open-Ended Marriage and Alternative Lifestyles*, 2nd ed. (Lincoln, Neb.: iUniverse, 2000), 17.
8. Interview with Wagner, August 6, 2007.

Chapter 6

1. Patti Thomas, *Recreational Sex: An Insider's Guide to the Swinging Lifestyle* (Cleveland: Peppermint Publishing Company, 2002), 14.
2. Terry Gould, *The Lifestyle: A Look at the Erotic Rites of Swingers* (Firefly Books, 2000), 10–11.

Chapter 7

1. Daphne Rose Kingma, *The Future of Love: The Power of the Soul in Intimate Relationships* (Broadway Books, 1998), 38.
2. Sarah Sloane, "Polyamory for Non-Primary Partners" workshop, Dark Odyssey, Washington, DC, December 2005.
3. Kingma, *The Future of Love*, 33.
4. Ibid., 147.

Chapter 9

1. Although a V triad that includes both sexes is technically either polygyny or polyandry, those terms are more often used by academics, rarely by polyamorous people themselves.
2. All these terms except *pod* were used by the people I interviewed. *Pod* was coined by Dr. Sasha Lessin and Janet Lessin to describe their multiperson polyamorous group (whose members were known as *podners*), and the term has gained some use and popularity in recent years among groups on the West Coast and in Hawaii.
3. Raven Kaldera, *Pagan Polyamory: Becoming a Tribe of Hearts* (Woodbury, Minn.: Llewellyn, 2005), 16.
4. Larry L. Constantine and Joan M. Constantine, *Group Marriage: A Study of Contemporary Multilateral Marriage* (Macmillan, 1973), 128.
5. Kaldera, *Pagan Polyamory*, 8.
6. E. S. Craighill Handy and Mary Kawena Pukui, cited in Deborah Taj-Anapol, "A Glimpse of Harmony," *Plural Loves: Designs for Bi and Poly Living*, Serena Anderlini-D'Onofrio, ed. (Harrington Park Press, 2004), 115.

Chapter 11

1. *Pansexual (also: polysexual, omnisexual)*: attraction to, having sex with, loving, and forming relationships with people of all genders. The term is also used to describe organizations or events that welcome people of all sexual orientations.

2. Gender activists promote the use of *ze* as the alternative for "he" and "she" and *hir* as the alternative for "him" and "her," "his" and "hers."

Chapter 12

1. David P. Barash and Judith Eve Lipton, *The Myth of Monogamy: Fidelity and Infidelity in Animals and People* (Henry Holt, 2001), 134.

2. Alison Rowan, "How to Be Not Monogamous," *Breaking the Barriers to Desire: New Approaches to Multiple Relationships*, Kevin Lano and Claire Parry, eds. (Five Leaves Publications, 1995), 17.

3. Raven Kaldera, *Pagan Polyamory: Becoming a Tribe of Hearts* (Woodbury, Minn.: Llewellyn, 2005), 41.

Chapter 13

1. "Compersion," Urban Dictionary, http://www.urbandictionary.com/define.php?term=compersion.

2. "Compersion," Polyamory Society, http://www.polyamorysociety.org/compersion.html.

3. "Compersion," Poly Oz, http://polyoz.dhs.org/component/option,com_rd_glossary/task,showcat/catid,37/Itemid,41/.

4. Raven Kaldera, *Pagan Polyamory: Becoming a Tribe of Hearts* (Woodbury, Minn.: Llewellyn, 2005), 77.

5. Serena Anderlini-D'Onofrio, "Plural Loves: Bi and Poly Utopias for a New Millennium," in *Plural Loves: Designs for Bi and Poly Living*, Serena Anderlini-D'Onofrio, ed. (Harrington Park Press, 2004), 4.

6. Eric Francis, "A Crazy Little Thing Called... ," Planet Waves, http://planetwaves.net/compersion.html.

Chapter 14

1. Dorothy Tennov, *Love and Limerence: The Experience of Being in Love*, 2nd ed. (Lanham, Md.: Scarborough House, 1999), 23–24.
2. Some people define NRE as "new relationship excitement"; it's the same concept.
3. Zhahai Stewart, "What's All This NRE Stuff, Anyway: Reflections 15 Years Later," *Loving More* no. 26 (2001), http://www.aphroweb.net/articles/nre.htm.
4. Raven Kaldera, *Pagan Polyamory: Becoming a Tribe of Hearts* (Woodbury, Minn.: Llewellyn, 2005), 50.
5. Geri D. Weitzman, "What Psychology Professionals Should Know About Polyamory," March 1999, http://www.polyamory.org/~joe/polypaper.htm.

Chapter 15

1. Daphne Rose Kingma, *The Future of Love: The Power of the Soul in Intimate Relationships* (Broadway Books, 1998), 12.
2. Amity Pierce Buxton, "Works in Progress: How Mixed-Orientation Couples Maintain their Marriages after the Wives Come Out," *Journal of Bisexuality* vol. 4, No. 1/2 (2004): 79.
3. Joy Davidson, PhD, "Working with Polyamorous Clients in the Clinical Setting," *Electronic Journal of Human Sexuality*, vol. 5, April 16, 2002, http://www.ejhs.org/volume5/polyoutline.html.

Chapter 16

1. Larry L. Constantine and Joan M. Constantine, *Group Marriage: A Study of Contemporary Multilateral Marriage* (Macmillan, 1973), 24–25.

Chapter 17

1. Valerie White, "Thinking About Children," *Loving More* no. 37 (Winter 2007), 12.

2. J. Watson and M. A. Watson, "Children of Open Marriages: Parental Disclosure and Perspectives," *Alternative Lifestyles* 5(1), 1982, 54–62, cited in Geri D. Weitzman, "What Psychology Professionals Should Know About Polyamory," www.polyamory.org/~joe/polypaper.htm, March 1999.

3. John Ullman, "Poly Parents: Talk Straight to Your Kids Even If It Scares the Bejesus Out of You," *Loving More* no. 37 (Winter 2007), 5.

4. Larry L. Constantine and Joan M. Constantine, *Group Marriage: A Study of Contemporary Multilateral Marriage* (Macmillan, 1973), 92.

5. Maria Pallotta-Chiarolli, "Poly Parents: Having Children, Raising Children, Schooling Children," *Loving More* no. 31 (Fall 2002), 8–12.

6. Arlene Istar Lev, LCSW, in *Proud Parenting*, quoted in White, "Thinking About Children," 13.

Chapter 18

1. Jon Knowles, "Chlamydia," rev. Jennifer Johnsen (March 2004), plannedparenthood.org.

2. Planned Parenthood Federation of America, "HPV," September 1, 2005, rev. June 28, 2007, http://www.plannedparenthood.org/sexual-health/std/hpv.htm.

3. Jon Knowles, "Genital Herpes" (1989), rev. Jennifer Johnsen and Jessica Davis (December 2004), plannedparenthood.org.

4. International Herpes Resource Center, "Safer Sex Tips," March 22, 2007, http://www.herpesresourcecenter.com/mvf.html.

5. Melissa Palmer, MD, *Dr. Palmer's Guide to Hepatitis and Liver Disease* (Avery, 2004), 82; Hepatitis Foundation International, hepfi.org.

6. Palmer, 92, 93; Danielle Dimitrov, "Hepatitis B" (February 2004), plannedparenthood.org; Hepatitis Foundation International, hepfi.org.

7. Palmer, 114.

8. Gay Men's Health Crisis, "Geffen Testing Center's HIV, Syphilis, and Hepatitis C Information Sheet,"
http://www.gmhc.org/health/testing/geffen_sti.html.

9. Palmer, 114; Hepatitis Foundation International, www.hepfi.org.

10. Gay Men's Health Crisis, "HIV & STI Testing,"
http://www.gmhc.org/health/testing.html.

Chapter 19

1. This quote and all others in the chapter are from my personal interview with Valerie White, August 9, 2007.

Chapter 20

1. Daphne Rose Kingma, *The Future of Love: The Power of The Soul in Intimate Relationships* (Broadway Books, 1998), 6.

Resource Guide

Every effort has been made to include the most current information. For updates to these lists and for a complete bibliography, see the *Opening Up* website, OpeningUp.net.

Books

Against Love, by Laura Kipnis (New York: Pantheon Books, 2003).

Anatomy of Love: The Natural History of Monogamy, Adultery and Divorce, by Helen Fisher (W. W. Norton, 1992).

Beyond Monogamy: Recent Studies of Sexual Alternatives in Marriage, edited by James R. Smith and Lynn G. Smith (Johns Hopkins University Press, 1974).

Bisexual and Gay Husbands: Their Stories, Their Words, edited by Fritz Klein and Thomas Schwartz (Binghamton, N.Y.: Harrington Park Press, 2001).

Breaking the Barriers to Desire: New Approaches to Multiple Relationships, edited by Kevin Lano and Claire Parry (Five Leaves Publications, 1995).

Compersion: Meditations on Using Jealousy as a Path to Unconditional Love (e-book), by Deborah Anapol (lovewithoutlimits.com, 2005).

Estate Planning for Same-Sex Couples, by Joan M. Burda (American Bar Association, 2004).

The Ethical Slut: A Guide to Infinite Sexual Possibilities, by Dossie Easton and Catherine A. Liszt (Oakland, Calif.: Greenery Press, 1998).

The Future of Love: The Power of the Soul in Intimate Relationships, by Daphne Rose Kingma (Broadway Books, 1998).

Group Marriage: A Study of Contemporary Multilateral Marriage, by Larry L. Constantine and Joan M. Constantine (Macmillan Publishing Company, 1973).

A Legal Guide for Lesbian & Gay Couples, by Denis Clifford, Frederick Hertz, and Emily Doskow (Nolo, 2007).

The Lesbian Polyamory Reader: Open Relationships, Non-Monogamy, and Casual Sex, edited by Marcia Munson and Judith P. Stelboum (Binghamton, N.Y.: Haworth Press, 1999).

Lesbian Polyfidelity: A Pleasure Guide for the Woman Whose Heart Is Open to Multiple, Concurrent Sexualoves, by Celeste West (San Francisco: Booklegger Publishing, 1996).

The Lifestyle: A Look at the Erotic Rites of Swingers, by Terry Gould (Richmond Hill, Ontario: Firefly Books, 2000).

Living Together: A Legal Guide for Unmarried Couples, by Ralph Warner, Toni Ihara, and Frederick Hertz (Nolo, 2006).

Loving More: The Polyfidelity Primer, by Ryam Nearing (Pep Publishing, 1992).

Mating in Captivity: Reconciling the Erotic and the Domestic, by Esther Perel (HarperCollins, 2006).

Money Without Matrimony: The Unmarried Couple's Guide to Financial Security, by Sheryl Garrett and Debra A. Neiman (Kaplan Business, 2005).

The Myth of Monogamy: Fidelity and Infidelity in Animals and People, 2nd ed., by David P. Barash and Judith Eve Lipton (Owl Books/Henry Holt, 2002).

The New Intimacy: Open-Ended Marriage and Alternative Lifestyles, by Ronald Mazur (Lincoln, Neb.: iUniverse, 2000).

Nonviolent Communication: A Language of Life, by Marshall B. Rosenberg (Encinitas, Calif.: PuddleDancer Press, 2003).

Open Marriage: A New Life Style for Couples, by Nena O'Neill and George O'Neill (M. Evans and Company, Inc., 1984).

Pagan Polyamory: Becoming a Tribe of Hearts, by Raven Kaldera (Woodbury, Minn.: Llewellyn Publications, 2005).

Plural Loves: Designs for Bi and Poly Living, edited by Serena Anderlini-D'Onofrio (Binghamton, N.Y.: Harrington Park Press, 2004).

Polyamory: Roadmaps for the Clueless & Hopeful, by Anthony D. Ravenscroft (Crookston, Minn.: Crossquarter Publishing Group, 2004).

Polyamory: The New Love Without Limits: Secrets of Sustainable Intimate Relationships, by Deborah M. Anapol (San Rafael, Calif.: Intinet Resource Center, 1997).

Recreational Sex: An Insider's Guide to the Swinging Lifestyle, by Patti Thomas (Cleveland, Ohio: Peppermint Publishing Company, 1997).

Redefining Our Relationships: Guidelines For Responsible Open Relationships by Wendy-O Matik (Oakland, Calif.: Defiant Times Press, 2002).

The Sex and Love Handbook: Polyamory! Bisexuality! Swingers! Spirituality! (& Even) Monogamy! A Practical Optimistic Relationship Guide, by Kris A. Heinlein and Rozz M. Heinlein (Do Things Records & Publishing, 2004).

Singled Out: How Singles are Stereotyped, Stigmatized, and Ignored, and Still Live Happily Ever After, by Bella DePaulo (St. Martin's Press, 2006).

Single State of the Union: Single Women Speak Out on the State of Life, Love, and the Pursuit of Happiness, edited by Diane Mapes (Seal Press, 2007).

Single: The Art of Being Satisfied, Fulfilled and Independent, by Judy Ford (Adams Media Corporation, 2004).

Swap Clubs: A Study in Contemporary Sexual Mores, by William and Jerrye Breedlove (Sherbourne Press, 1964).

Swinging for Beginners: An Introduction to the Lifestyle, by Kaye Bellemeade (New Tradition Books, 2003).

Swinging: Real Stories by Real Swingers, by Terry O'Day (Charleston, S.C.: BookSurge Publishing, 2005).

Three In Love: Ménages à Trois from Ancient to Modern Times, by Barbara Foster, Michael Foster, and Letha Hadady (Backinprint.com, 2000).

The Threesome Handbook: A Practical Guide to Sleeping with Three, by Vicki Vantoch (New York: Thunder's Mouth Press, 2007).

Unmarried to Each Other: The Essential Guide to Living Together as an Unmarried Couple, by Dorian Solot and Marshall Miller (Marlowe & Company, 2002).

Why We Love: The Nature and Chemistry of Romantic Love, by Helen Fisher (Owl Books, 2004).

Conferences and Events

Dark Odyssey (Washington, D.C., and Maryland)
    darkodyssey.com
Family Synergy Conference and Reunion (Los Angeles)
    familysynergy.org
Florida Poly Retreat (Brooksville, Fla.)
    Floridapolyretreat.com
Free Spirit Sacred Sexuality Beltane (Maryland)
    freespiritgathering.org/beltane
Heartland Polyamory Conference (French Lick, Ind.)
    heartlandpoly.com
Lifestyles Conventions
    lifestyles-conventions.com

Loving More Conferences and Retreats
    lovemore.com/conferences.shtm
NASCA Swinger Convention Listings
    nasca.com/states/nasca_convention.html
Naughty in N'awlins (New Orleans, La.)
    neworleansinnovember.com
Poly Big Fun (Bastrop, Tex.)
    Polybigfun.net
Poly Camp East (Seneca Rocks, W.V.)
    polycamp.net
Poly Camp Northwest (Bow, Wash.)
    polycamp.org
Poly Camp Ontario
    torontopoly.ca
PolyLiving Polyamory Conference (Philadelphia, Penn.)
    Polyliving.com
Swingfest (Florida)
    swingfest.com
Swingstock (Minneapolis)
    swingstock.com
World Polyamory Association West Coast Conference (Harbin Hot
Springs, Calif.)
    worldpolyamoryassociation.org

GLBT/Queer Resources

LGBT-Poly
    groups.yahoo.com/group/LGBT-Poly/
NYC Gay/Lesbian/Bi/Trans Polyamorists
    groups.yahoo.com/group/nyc-glbt-poly/
Polyamorous NYC (GLBT focus, GLBT-supportive folks welcome)
    poly-nyc.com

Local and Regional Organizations, Online Groups, Listservs, and Communities

UNITED STATES

Mid-Atlantic States

Chesapeake Polyamory Network, P.O. Box 5805, Takoma Park, MD 20913
    chespoly.org

Northwest

Inland NorthWest Poly (northern Idaho, Montana, and eastern Washington)
    groups.yahoo.com/group/INWPoly

Southeast

Polyamory Southeast (Alabama, Florida, Georgia, the Carolinas, and Tennessee)
    polysoutheast.org

Alabama

Alabama Polyamory
    groups.yahoo.com/group/alabamapolyamory/

Arizona

AZ Poly
    email azpoly-request@deepthot.org with "subscribe" in body of message
AZPolyP.U.R.P.O.S.E.
    groups.yahoo.com/group/AzPolyPurpose/
Liberated Christians, P.O. Box 32835, Phoenix, AZ 85064-2835
    libchrist.com
PolyTucson
    groups.yahoo.com/group/polytucson/

California

Bay Area Poly
  nakedunderleather.com/mailman/listinfo/bayareapoly
Berkeley Poly Women's Group
  polywog@goplay.com, 510-548-8283
Family Synergy
  P.O. Box 3073, Huntington Beach, CA 92605-3073
  familysynergy.org
Live The Dream
  8515 Penfield Avenue, Winnetka, CA 91406
  Live_TheDream2000@yahoo.com, 818-886-0069, ext. 3
Los Angeles Poly Support
  laps.org and groups.yahoo.com/group/losangelespolysupport/
North Bay Poly
  Announcements: groups.yahoo.com/group/north_bay_poly/
  Discussion: groups.yahoo.com/group/North_Bay_Poly_Chat/
Orange County Polyamory Network
  800-418-8202
Sacramento Polyamory Group
  groups.yahoo.com/group/sac-poly/community.livejournal.com/
  sac_poly/
San Diego Polyamory
  groups.yahoo.com/group/sandiegocaliforniapolyamory/
Santa Cruz Loving More
  Linda or Michael at 831-425-3448
Santa Cruz Polyamory
  groups.yahoo.com/group/santacruzpolyamory/
SoCalPoly
  groups.yahoo.com/group/SoCalPoly/
South Bay Polys
  P.O. Box 70203, Sunnyvale, CA 94086
  members.aol.com/wabaldwin/sbpolys.html

Connecticut

Connecticut Poly
> groups.yahoo.com/group/connecticut_polys/

Colorado

Squawk (Denver)
> To join the mailing list, send email to squawk-request@deepthot.org

Colorado Polyamory Community
> groups.yahoo.com/group/Colorado_Polyamory_Community/

Florida

Brevard Poly (Florida's Space Coast area)
> groups.yahoo.com/group/brevardpoly/

Pensacola Polyamory (Alabama/Florida Panhandle)
> groups.yahoo.com/group/Pensacola_Polyamory/

PolyCentral Florida (Orlando)
> polycentralfl.com and groups.yahoo.com/group/polycentral/

Poly Tampa
> polytampa.com

Georgia

Atlanta Poly
> polysoutheast.org/atlanta.html

Hawaii

Hawaiian Poly Pagans
> groups.yahoo.com/group/hi-polypagans/

Pali Paths—Honolulu Polyamory Network
> palipaths.org

Illinois

BiState Poly List (greater St. Louis metropolitan area, southwestern Illinois)
    groups.yahoo.com/group/BiStatePolyList/
Illinois Polyamory
    groups.yahoo.com/group/illinois_polyamory
PolyCU (Champaign/Urbana)
    shout.net/raul/polycu
PolyChi (Chicago)
    groups.yahoo.com/group/PolyChi/

Indiana

Fort Wayne Indiana Polyamory
    groups.yahoo.com/group/FortWayneIndianaPolyamory/
in-poly
    groups.yahoo.com/group/in-poly/

Iowa

Central Iowa Polyamory (Des Moines /Ames)
    groups.yahoo.com/group/centraliowapoly
Iowa Polyamory
    groups.yahoo.com/group/iowapolyamory/

Kansas

KanPoly
    kanpoly.org and groups.yahoo.com/group/KanPoly/
mopoly1 (Missouri and Kansas)
    groups.yahoo.com/group/mopoly1

Kentucky

KYPolyList—Kentucky Polyamory Community
    Discussion list: groups.yahoo.com/group/kypolylist
    Announcements list: groups.yahoo.com/group/KYPolyAnnounce
Polyamory of Central Kentucky (PoCK)
    groups.yahoo.com/group/PoCK

Maryland

Baltimore Maryland Polyamory Network
    groups.yahoo.com/group/BMPN/
Susquehanna Valley Polyamory Network (south-central Pennsylvania and northern Maryland)
    groups.yahoo.com/group/SVPN

Massachusetts

Family Tree
    P.O. Box 441275, Somerville, MA 02144
    ftree.contra.org
Poly-Boston
    To subscribe, send email with "subscribe" in the body of the message to: announce-request@boston.polyamory.org
    community.livejournal.com/polyboston/profile
Western Massachusetts Poly Events
    groups.yahoo.com/group/WMassPoly_Events/

Michigan

Metro Detroit Poly
    detroitmetropoly.com and groups.yahoo.com/group/det_polynet/
Michigan Polyamory Network
    groups.yahoo.com/group/michipoly/

Minnesota

PolyDuluth

    groups.yahoo.com/group/PolyDuluth/

PolyFargoMoorhead (Fargo, North Dakota, and Moorhead, Minnesota)

    groups.yahoo.com/group/PolyFargoMoorhead

PolyRochesterMN

    groups.yahoo.com/group/PolyRochesterMN

PolySaintCloudMN

    groups.yahoo.com/group/PolySaintCloudMN

Twin Cities Polyamory Discussion/Social/Support Group

    P.O. Box 240615, Apple Valley, MN 55124-0615

    mnpoly.org

Missouri

BiState Poly List (greater St. Louis metropolitan area, southwestern Illinois)

    groups.yahoo.com/group/BiStatePolyList/

mopoly1 (Missouri and Kansas)

    groups.yahoo.com/group/mopoly1

Montana

PburgPoly (Philipsburg)

    groups.yahoo.com/group/PburgPoly

Nebraska

Nebraska_Poly

    groups.yahoo.com/group/Nebraska_Poly

Nevada

PolyVegas

    groups.yahoo.com/group/PolyVegas

New Jersey

NJPoly

> groups.yahoo.com/group/njpoly/

New Mexico

New Mexico Polyamory Network

> nmpoly@twomoons.com

Albuquerque Poly Support Group

> nmpoly@yahoo.com

New York

Central New York Poly

> geocities.com/cnypoly

New York Gay/Lesbian/Bi/Transgender Polyamory

> groups.yahoo.com/group/nyc-glbt-poly

New York City Metro Area Polyamory List

> groups.yahoo.com/group/nyc-poly/

Polyamorous NYC (GLBT focus, GLBT-supportive folks welcome)

> poly-nyc.com

TriState Poly

> polyamory.org/~joe/nynj/ and groups.yahoo.com/group/nyc-poly/

North Carolina

NCPoly (Raleigh/Durham/Chapel Hill)

> openweave.org/NCPoly/

Triangle Polyamory Network (Durham)

> openweave.org/NCPoly/TPN.html

WNC/Asheville

> groups.yahoo.com/group/WNC-Poly/

North Dakota

PolyFargoMoorhead (Fargo, North Dakota, and Moorhead, Minnesota)
  groups.yahoo.com/group/PolyFargoMoorhead
PolyGrandForks
  groups.yahoo.com/group/PolyGrandForks

Ohio

Poly Columbus
  groups.yahoo.com/group/polycolumbus
Third Party Ohio
  groups.yahoo.com/group/ThirdPartyOhio

Oklahoma

OKPoly
  groups.yahoo.com/group/OKPoly

Oregon

Corvallis Polyamory Resource
  lm_ls@hotmail.com
NW_POLY_BDSM (Pacific Northwest)
  groups.yahoo.com/group/NW_POLY_BDSM
pdx-poly (Portland)
  groups.yahoo.com/group/PDX-POLY
Portland Crackers
  owner-crackers@polyrose.org
Portland Polyamory
  groups.yahoo.com/group/portlandpolyamory/

Pennsylvania

Central Pennsylvania Interracial Polyamory
    groups.yahoo.com/group/CentralPenn-Interracial-Poly
Philadelphia Mindful Polyamory Meetup Group
    polyamory.meetup.com/369/
Philly-Poly
    groups.yahoo.com/group/philly-poly/
Three Rivers Polyamory Network (Pittsburgh area)
    www.geocities.com/WestHollywood/Park/9573
Susquehanna Valley Polyamory Network (south-central Pennsylvania
and northern Maryland)
    groups.yahoo.com/group/SVPN

South Dakota

PolySiouxFalls
    groups.yahoo.com/group/PolySiouxFalls

Tennessee

TNPoly
    groups.yahoo.com/group/tnpoly

Texas

DFW-Poly (Dallas/Fort Worth)
    groups.yahoo.com/group/DFW-Poly
Poly-Austin
    groups.yahoo.com/group/poly-austin
Poly-Houston
    lists.polyamory.org/listinfo.cgi/poly-houston-polyamory.org
Poly-Texas
    grou.ps/poly_texas

Utah

Utah Polyamory Society
> groups.yahoo.com/group/UtahPolyamorySociety/

Vermont

Green Without Envy, The Vermont Poly Group
> Contact CaroleAM@hotmail.com

Virginia

Polyamory Virginia
> groups.yahoo.com/group/Polyamory_Virginia

Hampton Roads Polyamory (HaRP)
> hrpolyamory.com and groups.yahoo.com/group/harp

Roanoke Poly
> groups.yahoo.com/group/RoanokePoly

VA Poly Personals
> groups.yahoo.com/group/VAPolyPersonals

Washington

Center for Sex Positive Culture (Seattle)
> sexpositiveculture.org

Kitsap Poly
> groups.yahoo.com/group/KitsapPoly

Les-Bi-Poly (Seattle)
> groups.yahoo.com/group/Les-Bi-Poly

NW_Poly_BDSM (Pacific Northwest)
> groups.yahoo.com/group/NW_POLY_BDSM

Poly ForUUm of Greater Seattle (local chapter of Unitarian Universalists
for Polyamory Awareness)
> erosong.net/PolyForUUm.htm

Poly-in-Seattle
> groups.yahoo.com/group/poly-in-seattle

Sea-Poly
>   groups.yahoo.com/group/sea-poly

Seattle/Bellevue WA Weekly Poly Chat
>   emo123456789@juno.com

Seattle Poly Intimacy Network (SPIN)
>   wuzzle.org/~spin

Seattle Poly Potlucks
>   scn.org/~spg/index.html and groups.yahoo.com/group/Seattle-Poly-Potluck

Tac-Oly Poly (Tacoma/Olympia)
>   groups.yahoo.com/group/Tac-OlyPoly

Wisconsin

Polyamory in Wisconsin
>   groups.yahoo.com/group/Polyamory_In_Wisconsin

INTERNATIONAL

Canada

Atlantic Canada Polyamory
>   yahoogroups.com/subscribe/atlanticpoly

Bi-Polyamory-Ottawa
>   groups.yahoo.com/group/Bi-Polyamory-Ottawa

Polyamory Canada
>   yahoogroups.com/subscribe/polyamorycanada

Polyamory Newfoundland
>   groups.yahoo.com/group/polynfld

Polyamory Quebec
>   groups.yahoo.com/group/quebecpoly

Tobermory (Ontario) Poly
>   groups.yahoo.com/group/polytobermory

Toronto-Poly
>   yahoogroups.com/subscribe/TorontoPoly

Toronto Ontario Polys
>   groups.yahoo.com/group/toronto_ontario_polys

Vancouver Polyamory Group
>   groups.yahoo.com/group/vanpoly

Winnipeg Polyamory Discussion Group
>   yahoogroups.com/subscribe/win-poly

Mexico

Comunidad Polyamory De Mexico
>   polyamorymex.8m.com/

Europe

Polyamorous Europe
>   tribes.tribe.net/polyeurope

Austria

Polyamory Austria
>   yahoogroups.com/subscribe/polyamoryat

Denmark

Polydan
>   polydan.dk

France

Polyamour Network of Southern France
>   polyamour.net

Germany

Zegg (An Intentional Community)
>   zegg.de

Ireland

IE Poly
> pir.net/mailman/listinfo.cgi/iepoly

Netherlands

Polyamory Netherlands
> polyamory.nl

Portugal

Poly Portugal
> groups.yahoo.com/group/poly_portugal

Poliamor
> poliamor.pt.to

Spain

Poliamor Yahoo Group
> es.groups.yahoo.com/group/poliamor

Switzerland

Resource Center of Swiss Polyamory
> polyamory.ch

United Kingdom

Polyday
> polyday.org.uk

Scotland Based Polyamorists
> groups.yahoo.com/group/scots-poly

UK-POLY
> uk-poly.net

UK-poly
> bi.org/uk-poly

South Africa

Durban Polyamory
  groups.yahoo.com/group/durbanpoly
Polyamory South Africa
  freewebs.com/polyamory/home.htm

Australia

Australian Polyamory Network
  groups.yahoo.com/group/polyamory-australia
Polyamory Queensland
  groups.msn.com/PolyamoryQueensland
PolyOz: Polyamory Resources Australia
  polyoz.org
Poly Pioneers in Australia and New Zealand
  polypagan.tripod.com

New Zealand

Nelson Polyamory Society
  geocities.com/nz_polyamory/nelson.html
New Zealand Polyamory Group
  nzpoly.org.nz
Polyamory Wellington
  polyamory.org.nz
Poly Kiwis
  groups.yahoo.com/group/PolyKiwis
Poly Pioneers in Australia and New Zealand
  polypagan.tripod.com

Phillipines

Bi The Way
  groups.yahoo.com/group/bitheway

Magazines

Loving More
P.O. Box 4358, Boulder, CO 80306-4358
lovemore.com

National Organizations

The Alternatives to Marriage Project
    P.O. Box 320151, Brooklyn, NY 11232
    unmarried.org, 718-788-1911
Black Swingers Alliance
    blackswingersalliance.com
Human Awareness Institute
    hai.org
The Institute for 21st Century Relationships
    2419 Little Current Drive, Suite 1933, Herndon, VA 20171
    lovethatworks.org, 703-401-7230
International Lifestyle Association (Swinger Business Organization)
    theila.org
Loving More
    P.O. Box 4358, Boulder, CO 80306-4358
    lovemore.com, 303-543-7540
NASCA International (Swinger Business Organization)
    P.O. Box 7128, Buena Park, CA 90622-7128
    nasca.com
The National Coalition for Sexual Freedom
    822 Guilford Avenue, Box 127, Baltimore, MD 21202-3707
    ncsfreedom.org, 410-539-4824
Polyamory Society
    polyamorysociety.org

Sexual Freedom Legal Defense and Education Fund
    156 Massapoag Avenue, Sharon, MA 02067
    sfdlef.org, 781-784-6114
Woodhull Freedom Foundation
    1325 Massachusetts Avenue, NW, Suite 700, Washington, DC 20008
    woodhullfoundation.org, 202-628-3333
The World Polyamory Association
    The Lemurian Center, 2138 Vineyard Street, Wailuku, Hawaii 96793
    worldpolyamoryassociation.org, 808-244-4921, 808-244-4103

Online Groups and Lists

BD-SM Poly
    groups.yahoo.com/group/BD-SMPoly/
CPN Poly/Mono
    For polyamorous people with monogamous partners.
    groups.yahoo.com/group/cpnpolymono/
Domsub_Polyamory
    For those involved or interested in polyamorous D/s, BDSM, and
    Master/slave relationships.
    groups.yahoo.com/group/Domsub_Polyamory/
LiveJournal Polyamory Community
    community.livejournal.com/polyamory/
LovingMore LoveList
    groups.yahoo.com/group/LovingMore_lovelist/
Poly-Amory
    groups.yahoo.com/group/poly-amory/
Poly/Mono
    For monogamous people with polyamorous partners.
    groups.yahoo.com/group/PolyMono/
Polyamory Relationships
    groups.yahoo.com/group/PolyamoryRelationships/

Polyfamilies

> For people who are, have been, or wish to be in a polyamorous
> family of three or more adults (with or without children).
> groups.yahoo.com/group/polyfamilies/
> polyfamilies.com

Polyfidelity2

> For those who practice or hope to practice polyfidelity.   .
> groups.yahoo.com/group/polyfidelity2/

Poly-Thinkers

> For individualists, Heinleiners, people who are politically incorrect
> and unafraid of offending or being offended.
> groups.yahoo.com/group/poly-thinkers/

Women of Polyamory

> groups.yahoo.com/group/Women_of_Polyamory

Professional Directories

Resources for finding a therapist or other health care professional who
is informed about alternative sexualities and lifestyles.

American Association of Sexuality Educators, Counselors and Therapists
(AASECT)

> aasect.org

Bisexuality-Aware Professionals Directory

> List of professionals who are sensitive to the unique needs of a
> bisexual clientele.
> bizone.org/bap/

Kink-Aware Professionals

>   Resource for people seeking psychotherapeutic, medical, and legal
>   professionals who are informed about the diversity of consensual,
>   adult sexuality (maintained by the National Coalition for Sexual
>   Freedom).
>
>   ncsfreedom.org/index.php?option=com_keyword&id=270

Kink-Aware Professionals—Canada

>   kap.vancouverleather.com

Poly-Friendly Professionals

>   List of professionals who have been referred as or who have iden-
>   tified themselves as being open-minded about polyamory and
>   polyamorous issues.
>
>   polychromatic.com/pfp/

Opening Up Poly-Friendly Professionals Directory

>   Openingup.net

Research and Activism

Community-Academic Consortium for Research on Alternative Sexualities
(CARAS)

>   caras.ws

The Electronic Journal of Human Sexuality

>   Academic material on polyamory.
>
>   ejhs.org

Love and Politics

>   Organization for integrating polyamorous, queer, or sex-positive
>   identity into an overall vision for progressive change.
>
>   loveandpolitics.org
>
>   groups.yahoo.com/group/LoveAndPolitics/

LovingMore Polyactive

>   Political or activist issues relevant to polyamory.
>
>   groups.yahoo.com/group/LovingMorePolyactive/

PolyGreens

> Poly people interested in organizing within the Green Party.
> groups.yahoo.com/group/polygreens/

Polyleaders: Poly Leaders Network

> Discussion among poly activists and leaders on nurturing the polyamory movement and securing legal rights and protections for polyamorous relationships.
> groups.yahoo.com/group/polyleaders/

PolyModerators

> For coordinators of polygroups and polylists and those who wish to start a poly group.
> groups.yahoo.com/group/PolyModerators/

PolyResearchers

> People involved or interested in the academic research of polyamory.
> groups.yahoo.com/group/PolyResearchers/

Saturnia Regna

> Responsible nonmonogamous relationships and polyactivism.
> groups.yahoo.com/group/Saturnia_Regna/

Spirituality Resources

AhavaRaba

> Email list for people who are polyamorous and Jewish.
> commonhouse.net/mailman/listinfo/ahavaraba

Dark Odyssey

> An event that brings together BDSM, sexuality, spirituality, education, and play in a fun, supportive, nonjudgmental, diverse environment.
> darkodyssey.com

Free Spirit Sacred Sexuality Beltane

> freespiritgathering.org/beltane/

Poly Atheists (LiveJournal)

    community.livejournal.com/poly_atheists/

Poly Thinkers in Alternative Religions

    For polyamorists who are adherents of nonmainstream religions
    and spiritualities.

    groups.yahoo.com/group/poly-alt-religion-thinkers/

    angelfire.com/ny5/dvera/dv/poly/

Spiritual Polyamory

    Discussion list for those interested in polyamory and spirituality.

    groups.yahoo.com/group/spiritualpolyamory/

Unitarian Universalists for Polyamory Awareness

    uupa.org

Websites

Alt.Polyamory

    One of the very first online, resource-rich polyamory communities.

    polyamory.org

Franklin Veaux's Polyamory Info Page

    xeromag.com/fvpoly.html

Polyamory in the Media

    A great place to find out what's being written about polyamory in
    the media.

    polyinthemedia.blogspot.com

Polyamory Meetup Groups

    Meetup.com has been a boon to helping polyamorists connect
    and meet in real time. To find out if there is a polyamory meetup
    in your town, or to start one, go to polyamory.meetup.com and
    type in your ZIP code.

Polyamorous Percolations

>Strives to provide a comprehensive resource for people actively living in, curious about, or affected by a polyamorous relationship. polyamoryonline.org

Practical Polyamory

>Website of polyamory activist and educator Anita Wagner. Includes downloadable documents with in-depth content on dealing with polyamory relationship issues. practicalpolyamory.com

About the Interviewees

All questions on the questionnaire were open-ended—that is, there were no answers/categories to choose from—with one exception ("How would you describe your relationship style?").

Age
Average age (mean): 37*
Median age: 35
Most common age (mode): 32 and 43

AGE GROUP	NUMBER	PERCENTAGE
20–29	32	25%
30–39	55	44%
40–49	22	17%
50–59	13	10%
60–69	2	2%
70–79	2	2%

*Note: Of 126 respondents, four provided only a decade (e.g., "30s"). They are included in the age group data but not in the mean, median, and mode calculations.

Gender

GENDER	NUMBER	PERCENTAGE
Female	66	52%
Male*	50	40%
Transgender and Other**	10	8%

*Three men also identified as crossdressers.
**Includes MTF, FTM, trans, trans-entity, and gender neutral

Sexual Orientation

ORIENTATION	NUMBER	PERCENTAGE
Bisexual (includes bi, bi/queer, bi/pan, bi/straight)	48	38%
Straight (includes straight and straight/bi)	47	37%
Gay/lesbian/queer	24	19%
Pansexual/omnisexual	7	6%

BDSM Preference

PREFERENCE	NUMBER	PERCENTAGE
Kinky	64	51%
Not kinky	62	49%

Disability

RESPONSE	NUMBER	PERCENTAGE
Disabled	8	6%
Not disabled	118	94%

Race and Ethnicity

RACE/ETHNICITY	NUMBER	PERCENTAGE [of those who gave a response]
African American	6	5%
Asian American	4	3%
Caucasian	95	77%
Caucasian/Jewish	6	5%
Latino/a	4	3%
Native American	1	1%
Other*	7	6%
No response	3	

*Includes the following responses: Latino/African American, Caucasian/Israeli, Caucasian/Latino, Indian/Caucasian, "Very mixed"

Relationship Style

STYLE	NUMBER*	PERCENTAGE*
Monogamous	12	10%
Nonmonogamous	19	15%
Open relationship	20	16%
Polyamorous	68	54%
Polyfidelitous	10	8%
Swinger	9	7%
Other	6	5%

*Numbers do not total 100 and percentages do not total 100%; some respondents chose more than one style.

Primary Relationships

(Responses to the question "Do you consider one relationship primary?")

RESPONSE	NUMBER	PERCENTAGE [of those who gave a response]
Yes—one primary	78	68%
No	8	7%
No—two primaries	13	11%
No—three primaries	1	1%
No—don't believe in primary or hierarchy	14	12%
No response	4	
Not applicable	8	

Marriage

RESPONSE	NUMBER	PERCENTAGE [of those who gave a response]
Legally married to one partner	53	43%
Engaged to marry one partner	4	3%
Unmarried	67	54%
No response	2	

Out about Relationship Style

WHO	NUMBER*	PERCENTAGE* [of those who gave a response]
Out to everyone	26	22%
All friends	87	74%
Selected friends	28	24%
A few friends	3	3%
All family	50	42%
Selected family	34	29%
All co-workers	34	29%
Selected co-workers	24	20%
No response	8	

*Numbers do not total 100 and percentages do not total 100%; some respondents included more than one category in a response (e.g., "I am out to all my friends and select family members.")

Children

STATUS	NUMBER	PERCENTAGE [of those who gave a response]
With children	50	40%
Without children	74	60%
No response	2	

Out to Children

(Responses to the question "Are you out to your children about your
nonmonogamy/polyamory/open relationship?" by the 50 respondents
who reported they had children)

STATUS	NUMBER	PERCENTAGE [of those who gave a response]
Out to all children	25	52%
Out to older children only	5	11%
Not out because children are too young	3	6%
Not out	15	31%
No response	2	

Geography
(US Census Regions)

REGION	NUMBER	PERCENTAGE
West (AZ, CA, CO, OR, WA)	25	20%
Midwest (IA, IL, IN, KS, MI, MN, MO, OH, WI)	24	19%
South (AL, DC, FL, GA, MD, NC, OK, TX, VA)	38	30%
Northeast (CT, MA, NJ, NY, PA)	37	29%
Canada	2	2%

Occupation

(Categories from the Standard Occupational Classification (SOC) system
of the US Department of Labor, Bureau of Labor Statistics)
Note: The occupation most often named was "teacher" (6).

OCCUPATION	NUMBER	PERCENTAGE
Management	5	4%
Business and financial operations	8	6%
Computer and mathematical	12	9%
Architecture and engineering	3	2%
Life, physical, and social sciences	5	4%
Community and social services	9	7%
Legal	3	2%
Education, training, library	10	8%
Arts, design, entertainment, sports, and media	25	20%
Health care practitioners and practical occupations	1	1%
Health care support	3	2%
Food preparation and service	1	1%
Building and grounds cleaning and maintenance	1	1%
Sales and related occupations	5	4%
Office and administrative support	13	10%
Construction and extraction	1	1%
Installation, maintenance, and repair	1	1%
Military (enlisted)	1	1%
Homemaker	3	2%
Student	4	3%
Other*	8	6%
No response	2	2%

*Responses not specific enough to be classified

About the Author

TRISTAN TAORMINO is an award-winning author, columnist, editor, and sex educator. She is the author of *True Lust: Adventures in Sex, Porn and Perversion*; *Down and Dirty Sex Secrets*; and *The Ultimate Guide to Anal Sex for Women* and editor of the Lambda Literary Award–winning anthology series *Best Lesbian Erotica*. She is a columnist for the *Village Voice* and *Hustler's Taboo*. She runs her own adult film production company, Smart Ass Productions, and is currently an exclusive director for Vivid Entertainment. For Vivid, she directs the reality series *Chemistry*, winner of several awards, including the 2007 AVN Award for Best Gonzo Release. She also helms Vivid's sex education imprint, Vivid-Ed, for which she has written, produced, and directed four titles: *The Expert Guide to Anal Sex*; *The Expert Guide to Oral Sex 1: Cunnilingus*; *The Expert Guide to Oral Sex 2: Fellatio*; and *The Expert Guide to the G-Spot*.

Tristan has been featured in over 250 publications including the *New York Times*, *Redbook*, *Cosmopolitan*, *Glamour*, *Entertainment Weekly*, *Details*, *New York Magazine*, *Men's Health*, and *Playboy*. She has appeared on HBO's *Real Sex*, *The Howard Stern Show*, *Loveline*, *Ricki Lake*, and on CNN, MTV, and The Discovery Channel. She lectures at top colleges and universities, where she speaks on gay and lesbian issues, sexuality and gender, alternative relationships, and feminism. She teaches sex and relationship workshops around the world and runs two websites, puckerup.com and openingup.net. She lives in upstate New York with her partner and their three dogs.